VEGAN INTERMITTENT FASTING

Lose Weight, Reduce Inflammation, and Live Longer—the 16:8 Way

PETRA BRACHT, MD AND MIRA FLATT

THE EXPERIMENT

NEW YORK

The Experiment, LLC
220 East 23rd Street, Suite 600
New York, NY 10010-4658
theexperimentpublishing.com

This book contains the opinions and ideas of its author. It is intended to provide helpful and informative material on the subjects addressed in the book. It is sold with the understanding that the author and publisher are not engaged in rendering medical, health, or any other kind of personal professional services in the book. The author and publisher specifically disclaim all responsibility for any liability, loss, or risk—personal or otherwise—that is incurred as a consequence, directly or indirectly, of the use and application of any of the contents of this book.

THE EXPERIMENT and its colophon are registered trademarks of The Experiment, LLC. Many of the designations used by manufacturers and sellers to distinguish their products are claimed as trademarks. Where those designations appear in this book and The Experiment was aware of a trademark claim, the designations have been capitalized.

The Experiment's books are available at special discounts when purchased in bulk for premiums and sales promotions as well as for fund-raising or educational use. For details, contact us at info@theexperimentpublishing.com.

Library of Congress Cataloging-in-Publication Data

Names: Bracht, Petra, author. | Flatt, Mira, author.
Title: Vegan intermittent fasting : lose weight, reduce inflammation, and
   live longer-the 16:8 way / Petra Bracht, MD, and Mira Flatt.
Other titles: Intervallfasten. English
Description: New York : The Experiment, 2020. | Originally published in
   Germany as Intervallfasten and Das Kochbuch zum Intervallfasten by
   GRÄFE UND UNZER VERLAG GmbH, München, in 2019.
Identifiers: LCCN 2020034605 (print) | LCCN 2020034606 (ebook) | ISBN
   9781615197286 (paperback) | ISBN 9781615197293 (ebook)
Subjects: LCSH: Reducing diets. | Reducing diets--Recipes. | Intermittent
   fasting. | Low-calorie diet--Recipes. | LCGFT: Cookbooks.
Classification: LCC RM222.2 .B6484 2020 (print) | LCC RM222.2 (ebook) |
   DDC 613.2/5--dc23
LC record available at https://lccn.loc.gov/2020034605
LC ebook record available at https://lccn.loc.gov/2020034606

ISBN 978-1-61519-728-6
Ebook ISBN 978-1-61519-729-3

Cover design by Beth Bugler
Text design by Sarah Schneider
Cover photograph by Stocksy
Author photographs by Katharina Werner
Text by Petra Bracht and Mira Flatt
Translated by Joseph Smith and Irmela Erckenbrech

Manufactured in China

First printing December 2020
10 9 8 7 6 5 4 3 2 1

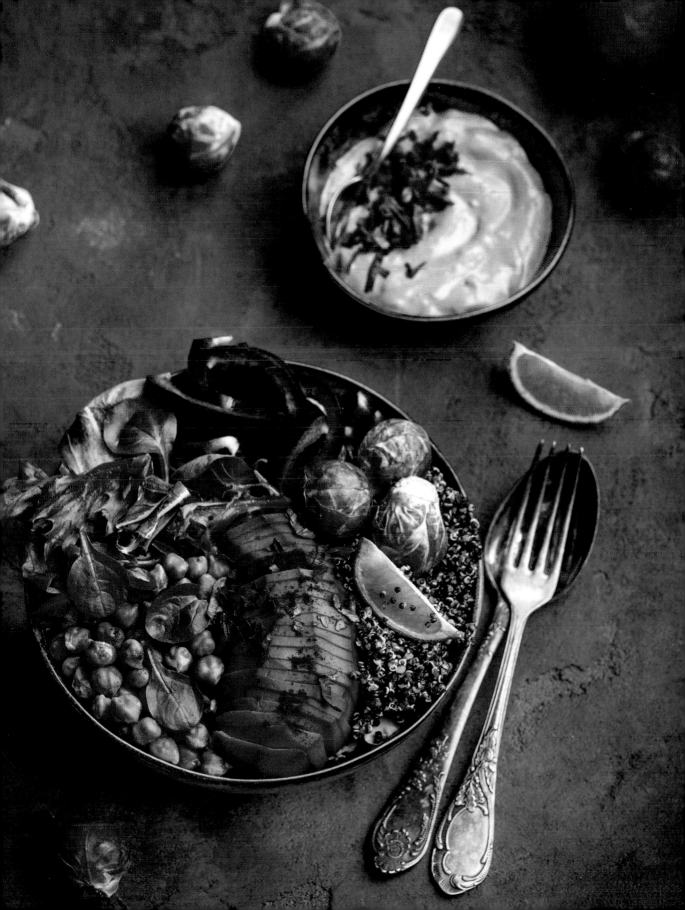

CONTENTS

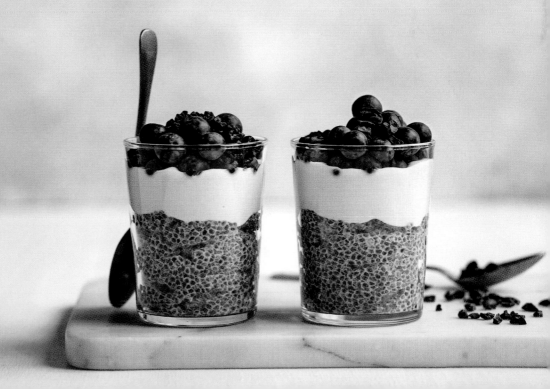

PREFACE

It was a very satisfying experience for me when the subject of intermittent fasting first started coming up in discussions of nutritional medicine. The knowledge and experience I had been accumulating over the years had finally been validated by expert and independent research. Finally, the media was paying attention to it, which of course makes my work with patients easier. And now, the long-winded discussions and skepticism are subsiding. Even my colleagues' aggressive comments have slowly died down—once they recognized how poor their knowledge of intermittent fasting had been.

Yet scientists tend to be reticent to celebrate these discoveries; there are, they claim, still not enough long-term studies available on human subjects. But they don't have my experience. My goal with this book is to present, in a way that everyone can understand, the amazing results that will convince even the greatest skeptics. Then, you can decide for yourself whether you should wait years before embarking on this journey. That's how long it will take until medical science, with its high standards for research, catches up and confirms the potential that my patients and I know lies in this method.

So, now it's up to you to apply these findings, as many of my patients have already done. I urge you to apply them *now*: You only have one chance to live in the body you've been given. I can guarantee that living the intermittent-fasting lifestyle will make for an exciting adventure—of that you can be certain!

Petra Bracht, MD

PART ONE

Intermittent Fasting

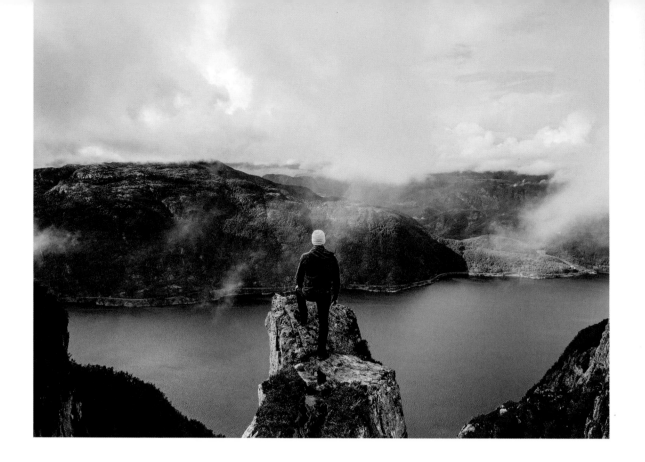

The Wonders of Fasting

Fasting is as old as humanity itself and is squarely anchored in our genes. It has amazing effects on our health and our life span. In fact, it's like a magic bullet. And maybe that's the reason it hasn't been completely forgotten over time, although it's become increasingly rare for people in the Western world to go hungry during hard times. Of course, fasting is also well known as a religious practice, in a number of different religions. Nevertheless, it remains a hotly debated topic. Proponents of natural healing have always been fans, but many conventional physicians still reject fasting as damaging to human health.

But times are changing—and thank goodness! The newest research results are causing quite a stir. Fasting today, especially intermittent fasting, has created so many possibilities for a healthy and long life.

I have used these advantages nearly all my life, albeit more intuitively than anything else. I've practiced intermittent fasting now for more than forty years. Why? Because it proved to be good for me. I began fasting without the knowledge of the amazing advantages it offers for a healthy lifestyle, which are now becoming clear to everyone. For the first ten years, I did this quietly, without much fanfare, since, at the time, failing to eat a hearty breakfast was considered a no-no, as was going to university lectures on an empty stomach and eating meals only twice (sometimes only once) a day.

However, I must admit, the quality of my diet wasn't optimal. Like most people at the time, I, too, consumed mainly the foods I was used to eating at home, including meat, among other things. I had never really liked drinking milk, but the omnipresent ads touting its positive effects for health led me to trick myself into drinking it. I made milkshakes and chocolate milk and ate lots of cheese, all to ensure sufficient milk intake.

This changed abruptly in 1991, when I was already a practicing primary care physician. I had been dissatisfied with conventional medicine for quite a while, and it was becoming clearer to me that what I had learned in my studies was not what I had once envisioned for myself as a doctor. What I wanted was to treat knowledgeable, empowered patients, whom I could lead to being healed. I hadn't become a physician just to suppress symptoms of diseases by prescribing medicines.

By chance, I came upon the book *Fit for Life* by Harvey and Marilyn Diamond, which changed my outlook on food and medicine. I devoured it in a few hours. Suddenly, it all became clear: Nutrition plays a key role in the prevention and healing of diseases. At the time, I failed to understand how that book would completely change my life and my career as a physician. It imparted to me the most important principles of *natural hygiene*, as it was then called, a health movement with the goal of *preventing* diseases through natural means.

The "Fit for Life" Movement

One of the most important tenets of the "Fit for Life" movement is based on the principle of natural bodily cycles, which states that we should consume food only between the hours of noon and 8:00 PM, so that it can be utilized by the body between 8:00 PM and 4:00 AM and then excreted between 4:00 AM and noon. Should this cycle be interrupted, say, by eating an early breakfast, then the waste materials would instead be deposited in the space between our cells (interstitial space) and in the connective tissue (fascia). This method also calls for significantly reducing the amount of meat and dairy products we consume. The main source of our diet should be fresh, plant-based foods.

My Greatest Discovery

I can still remember how excited I was. Finally—finally—I had discovered the reason why I had never felt hungry in the morning.

This was also around the time my husband and I decided to change our diet to include about 95 percent whole plant-based foods. What happened to us then can only be described as magnificent, prompting me to immediately incorporate nutritional medicine into my daily practice. Not all of my patients were happy about this move: It's so much easier for people with diabetes, high blood pressure, or gout, for example, to simply swallow a pill than to change their dietary habits!

Of course, every patient must make this decision for themselves. But those who let themselves be persuaded to take the more challenging path and try a change in diet to solve their underlying medical problems were, more often than not, rewarded with considerable improvement and, in some cases, complete healing.

Had I not been privy to these fantastic healing experiences myself, I would not have been able to continue down this path. But I've found that nearly all types of diseases react to fasting and proper nutrition. Once my patients had mentally prepared themselves for these changes, I began prescribing a fasting cure, as I was convinced of the potential of fasting therapy.

Intermittent Fasting: A Great Alternative to Long-Term Fasting

For many people, long-term fasting (see page 6) is hard to maintain. My husband, Roland, for example, was not a fan. One attempt he made turned out to be such torture for him that he quit after only five days. It was so surprising to me, because he's one of the most strong-willed people I know. But his body just couldn't take it, since, at the time, he was doing physical training for at least eight hours every day. Of course, he was upset with himself: He desperately wanted to enjoy all of the health advantages fasting could provide. So, imagine the relief he had at discovering intermittent fasting! He has since become a passionate fasting disciple.

What happened to him happened to many of my patients as well. Fasting for sixteen hours a day takes some getting used to at the beginning, but after ten days or so, the habit starts to set in. And being able to eat two to three times within a space of eight hours turns out to be a joy. You start to feel your hunger once again; things taste better, more intense; you can feel how your body becomes satiated; you feel empowered, whether at work or during physical activity. And, to boot, you start to lose that excess weight—and who wouldn't want that?

But there are even more advantages: Intermittent fasting is also the best way to prevent most lifestyle diseases. And if you already suffer from such a disease, you can expect your body to heal and become healthier over time. I have been blessed to have accompanied many of my patients during this process, and it's a joy to observe how much strength and energy intermittent fasting with a plant-based diet and the proper amount of physical exercise can instill in a human being.

Types of Fasting

LONG-TERM FASTING

Going without food for forty-two days is not an easy undertaking. But if you succeed in holding out, you'll be grateful you did. This method of fasting is often rooted in religious beliefs. It's said to bring one closer to God, to clear one's thoughts, and to purify the soul. All of the advantages of intermittent fasting can also be achieved through long-term fasting—but long-term fasting is much more difficult.

Fasting for six weeks changes the body—and the spirit—considerably, and both changes can be felt intensely. During this time, you are completely engaged with your body. You experience and work through any symptoms of illness directly; your feelings run rampant. Toward the end of the allotted fasting time, a sense of order returns to the body: You feel reborn. It's also common for many changes to take place in your life afterward. I remember one patient who, after fasting, divorced her husband, quit her job, and left her religious community. Today, she still fasts occasionally, generally for five to seven days at a time, though she hasn't made any additional severe changes to her life.

THERAPEUTIC FASTING

This method of fasting is probably the most well known. It was introduced by the German physician Otto Buchinger in the nineteenth century. A fasting period generally lasts about five to seven days, though longer regimens of up to thirty days are also possible. During this time, one consumes a maximum of five hundred calories a day, in the form of diluted fruit and vegetable juices, and, when necessary, a little honey. This method also emphasizes purging the bowels with the use of Epsom salt or Glauber's salt. Even today, Buchinger fasting clinics are very popular in Europe and attract many spa guests who return year after year. The reason is clear: People who stick with this regimen feel better after fasting, both physically and mentally.

The advantages of therapeutic fasting in specialized clinics lie in the close medical supervision provided by experienced physicians and therapists. But, of course, staying at a clinic may not lie within everyone's budget. And no one should underestimate the stress that can be caused by fasting there for a few days or even weeks: It can negatively affect your mood, creativity, and vigor. You may also feel isolated during this time. You won't be able to maintain normal daily interactions initially, unless you happen to be fasting with like-minded people.

Therapeutic fasting is not recommended for normal daily life—it should only be done when taking a time-out from your daily routine. Remember, it's a gift that the advantages of therapeutic fasting can also be fully experienced using intermittent fasting, which allows you to eat your fill and does not force you to act against your natural instincts.

JUICE FASTING

This is actually one of my favorite types of fasting, which I practice once or twice a year in addition to intermittent fasting. It's very easy to make it part of your daily routine. Because you are allowed to drink two to three large juices or smoothies a day (preferably the green kind), you aren't left feeling hungry and can generally avoid the usual "crises" experienced in the first few days of a long-term fast. The first smoothie of the day should be sweet, the second and third more hearty, with lots of vegetables and less fruit. Also, by getting all the vital substances and fiber it needs, the body can safely expel waste materials and ensure the optimal state of the intestinal microbiota.

Today, this type of fasting may take place in many hotels or specialized country getaways, which provide an ideal atmosphere to practice it. It's also easy to keep to a regimen of daily exercise, including endurance and strength training as well as stretching, since juice fasting doesn't sap one's energy level but in fact raises it. Afterward, when you start or continue a normal intermittent fasting program, you'll discover that food tastes like ambrosia to you—and readjusting your whole lifestyle will come easily to you.

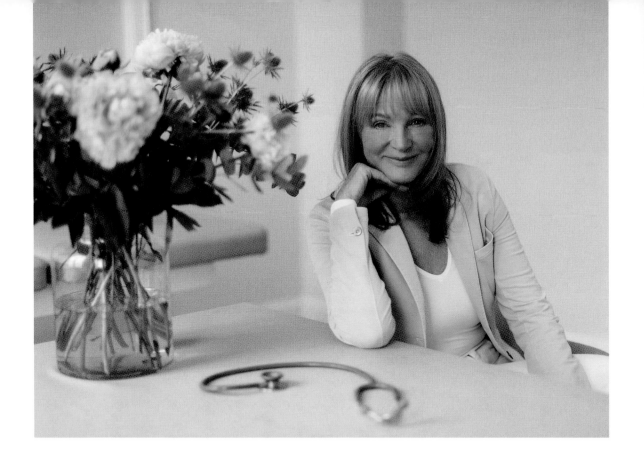

Refocusing Medicine

have worked as a general practitioner and natural health therapist for over thirty-five years. During this time, standard medical practice has changed considerably. There have never been so many different means of diagnosis available as there are today, as we can now gain such detailed knowledge about the state of a patient's blood, stool, and inner organs. Never before have we had so many

drugs, therapies, and medical technologies. And never before have so many extensive and complicated operations been carried out, so many organs replaced or biological functions supported by artificial means.

Mainstream medicine does amazing things. Even the most severe injuries can be "repaired" today, to the extent the patient can look forward to a bright future: The loss of limbs is remedied with artificial ones; artificial transducers are inserted to remedy hearing loss; technology takes over where biology fails. And that's only the beginning! In the future, biotechnology will surely be able to perform even greater miracles. That, in short, is the sunny side of modern high-tech, high-performance medicine, which no one—including myself—wants to do without.

At the same time, lifestyle diseases are increasing dramatically—and, more and more, they are happening in younger people. This includes cancer and circulatory diseases primarily, followed by autoimmune disorders, rheumatoid arthritis, type 2 diabetes, and fatty liver disease, which are largely caused by obesity. We are also seeing an increase in dementia, pain disorders, and damage to joints and the spine—not to mention a host of mental conditions like depression. All this *despite* the powers of modern medicine, which, it should be added, does attempt to remedy these conditions with medicines and operations.

The Limits of Conventional Medicine

It is paramount that we understand that any attempt to attack these diseases with drugs and operations cannot lead to true healing as long as the root causes— namely, poor nutrition and lack of physical movement—are not eliminated. Conventional high-performance medicine

desperately tries to alleviate the *symptoms* and the pain associated with the diseases. This derives from the false assumption that these methods serve the entire body. But is that true?

These medicines may target and correct certain symptoms of a disease, but at the same time they force the body out of balance. That's what you are reading about in the "Side Effects" pamphlet that comes with your medicine. And sometimes the side effects can be worse than the disease itself! But, as we know, these medicines don't root out the *cause* of a disease; they merely treat the symptoms.

So, What Is the Solution?

Conventional treatments can be effective at treating the symptoms, but not eliminating the causes, of the most common lifestyle diseases. For that purpose, we need natural, biologically appropriate approaches to actually resolve the source of the problem. The goal is to enable our powers of self-healing—what I call the "inner doctor"—that is, potent systems of self-regulation located in the genes of each and every human being, to enable our body to free itself of diseases on its own.

Activating Our Powers of Self-Healing

You can activate your own powers of self-healing naturally. And that doesn't mean taking drugs or undergoing surgery. It's simple: Avoid everything that would hinder your body from fulfilling its natural processes.

The Two Most Important Factors

According to studies done in the United States[1] and around the world,[2] life expectancy is now decreasing. It's becoming clear that our modern lifestyle is effectively shortening our life span. There are two factors that impede our innate powers of self-healing, leading to a variety of diseases, which usually occur before age fifty. Because our ability to self-heal is decreased, diseases can more easily spread and intensify throughout our body.

The first factor is nutrition. This is everything we put into our bodies on a daily basis in the form of foods and fluids. It seems logical that what we eat plays a major role in our health. What is not logical (and is actually alarming) is that, even today, the role of nutrition in health is hardly taught to medical students.

The second factor is physical activity. This, too, would seem to be a no-brainer: The human body functions better if it keeps moving. The simple idiom "If you rest, you rust" remains true today, but knowledge concerning physical activity plays only a minor role in the training of health-care personnel, regardless of medical specialty.

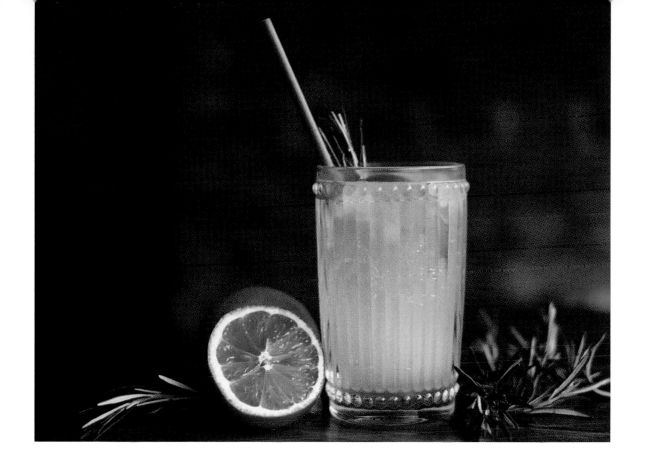

We Eat Too Much and Too Often

Forced fasting—fasting in times of scarcity—is hardwired into our genes. Historically, we ate what we could hunt and gather, meaning food wasn't always readily available. As a result, the body developed amazing survival mechanisms (see pages 15 to 26). When there was nothing or little to eat, our bodies went into survival mode, repairing and restoring itself at the cellular level. At the same time, fertility sank, meaning fewer children were born, to preserve what little food was available. When the food supply increased once again, the body resumed normal functioning and fertility rose, resulting in more offspring to ensure the survival of the species. Thus, times of sufficient food supply alternated with those of insufficient supply. Over the course of time, everything remained balanced.

The Underbelly of Life in the Land of Plenty

Today, modern Western nations have a significant food surplus. On one hand, that may seem to be a blessing, but it can actually be a major problem for our health. Because we are continually confronted with this excess food supply, we tend to eat more than we should—and for longer than we should.

Earlier suggestions that we should eat five (smaller) meals a day have been debunked.[3] Furthermore, modern humans no longer experience forced fasting, even though our bodies are still programmed to switch back and forth between states of eating and starving. The result is that the mechanisms that are set in motion when we starve—and that keep us healthy—no longer take place, leading to dramatic, in some cases health-shattering, consequences.

One serious result of a life without starvation phases is that many people suffer from, and even die of, diseases stemming from the consumption of too much food (and this is sometimes exacerbated by eating unhealthy foods) and drinking too much alcohol and sugary beverages. This situation is what I call the "dead-end of nutritional evolution." It is impossible to escape this dilemma if we do not very consciously face the reality of our excess food supply. And we must, since we know that a reduction in our food intake can in fact lengthen our life span (see page 13).

Why We Don't Want to Fast

Our ancestors never had to make a conscious decision concerning their food intake. If there was enough food available, they helped themselves to an extra portion—that was the easiest way to increase the probability that they would survive the next period of scarcity. If there was a dearth of food, they were forced to just live with it. That's why it is genetically and psychologically deeply ingrained in our bodies to fill our stomachs in times of bounty.

That may also be the reason why today we find it so hard to stop piling the food on our plates. Consciously and willfully starving goes against our instincts. And even when we have come to understand the problem, it doesn't actually solve the problem: Submitting ourselves to voluntary periods of starvation means overcoming innate obstacles each and every time.

Eat Less, Live Longer and Healthier

We have known for some time now from studies involving animals that a low-calorie diet serves to extend the life of the subjects without damaging their health and well-being.[4] But do these findings apply to human beings?

The Recent History of Fasting

The healing effect of fasting on certain diseases was first noted by the Greek doctor Hippocrates (ca. 460–370 BCE). Nearly two thousand years later, the Swiss-Austrian doctor and scholar Paracelsus (ca. 1493–1541 CE) tried to activate his "inner doctor" by limiting his food intake. Many early religious leaders, including the Buddha, Jesus, and Mohammed, practiced fasting as a means of attaining a higher level of consciousness. To this very day, major world religions, such as Christianity, Judaism, Hinduism, and Islam, include fasting as a fixed part of their belief system. The prescribed fasting periods of these religions still have positive effects on the health of the practicing believers.

Only in the nineteenth and later in the twentieth century did modern doctors such as Max Bircher-Benner (1867–1939), Otto Buchinger (1878–1966), and Franz Xaver Mayr (1875–1965) study fasting from a therapeutic point of view. This led to the creation of various fasting techniques, and the establishment of several clinics in Germany, Austria, and around the world. For example, Buchinger was the first to describe the physiology of fasting in his 1935 book *Das Heilfasten* (*About Fasting*); his technique, still implemented at the clinic he founded in 1920, advocates for fasting in conjunction with spirituality and community interaction. And the FX Mayr cure, which combines fasting with manual abdominal massages, continues to be implemented to this day at Mayr clinics around the world.

A Serendipitous Discovery, Thanks to Biosphere 2

Modern fasting research got a big boost from an accidental discovery. The US doctor and pathologist Roy Walford, a mentor of the cell biologist and gerontologist Valter Longo, had set the goal of using the Biosphere 2 project to prove that an ecosystem completely closed off from the outside world could be self-sufficient. But it failed: The oxygen supply dwindled to the point that it had to be supplemented from the outside. Further, vermin invaded the biosphere, which reduced the harvest of the fruits and vegetables within. But the scientists involved didn't quite want to give up. Instead, they simply ate less for the next two years. When the eight inhabitants eventually left the dome in the Arizona desert in 1991, they were emaciated and frustrated.

But a major surprise was in the offing when their medical exams took place. All of the former residents were in excellent health with optimal blood panels. In short, they were truly healthy. Their low cholesterol numbers were particularly striking, and this was doubly surprising since, according to conventional medicine, their diet should not have affected these numbers. As a result, Valter Longo dedicated himself to studying the effects of aging. Once, in an interview, he said that it wasn't the process of aging that interested him but actually the process of staying young.

Insulin-Like Growth Factor 1 (IGF-1)

Another groundbreaking discovery supports the healthy benefits of fasting. Dr. Jaime Guevara-Aguirre, a scientist and physician from Quito, Ecuador, studied a group of three hundred people with Laron syndrome, a congenital disease marked by the failure to generate insulin-like growth factor 1 (IGF-1) and the dysfunction of the liver's growth hormone receptor, leading to dwarfism. But what makes this disease especially fascinating is that the people suffering from Laron syndrome have an apparent ability to resist certain diseases. During Dr. Guevara-Aguirre's study period,

not a single person was afflicted by diabetes, and only one person developed cancer.[5]

John Kopchick (Ohio University) and Andrzej Bartke (Southern Illinois University) were able to prove that the life expectancy of mice could be extended by 40 percent if the IGF-1 receptors in their livers were turned off.[6] A normal IGF-1 value thus has a positive effect on growth and reproductivity, though it also shortens life and causes more disease when continually elevated.

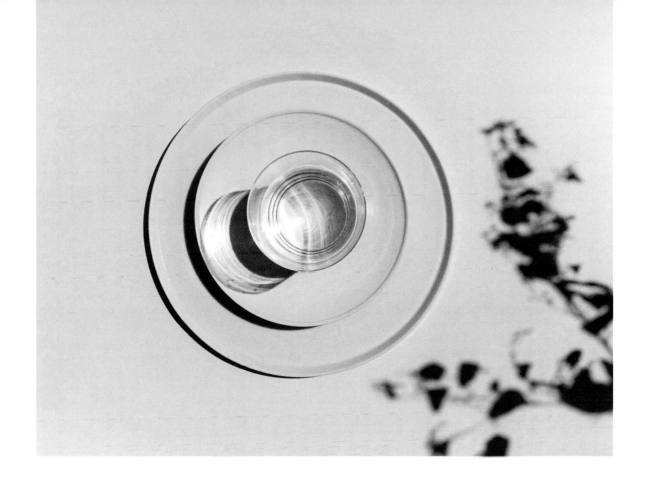

What Happens in the Body During Fasting

The results of scientific research you are about to learn are more than just impressive—they are revolutionary! Intermittent fasting is not just an important supplement to conventional medical treatment of various diseases—it is absolutely essential.

I'm so confident about this because of what I've observed in my patients over the past three decades: Again and again, I see how intermittent fasting, combined with a vegan diet and sufficient physical exercise, can literally make diseases "superfluous." People who have lived according to this method for long periods of time remain very healthy, which is why I am convinced that the method I suggest in this book will reduce your chance of getting ill to nearly zero.

If your doctors reject the idea of fasting, bring them the evidence and let them do the research. If they're even moderately open to new research, you may find that, in the end, they will renounce their prejudices. The newest scientific evidence proves even the most magnificent healing effects of fasting, something followers of natural medicine have observed for a very long time.

Autophagy: Recycling, Not Muscle Loss

Autophagy, the controlled self-digestion and reclamation of waste products in our cells and interstitial cell spaces, occurs during fasting periods. This naturally occurring recycling program is an ingenious function of our body. Its discovery by Japanese researcher Yoshinori Ohsumi earned him the Nobel Prize for Medicine in 2016. Frank Madeo at the University of Graz in Austria has also been looking into this phenomenon for many years now.

You can imagine what happens by envisioning the following: If you have been fasting for twelve hours, a waste-reduction squad makes its way to your cells, transporting loads of enzymes along with it. Not only does it then proceed to remove the waste materials in your body, but it also recycles these products. That's fascinating! In times of fasting, your body isn't replenished with new materials but must make do, using deposited cell waste to reproduce new and high-quality building materials. Imagine the bodily refuse being put in a compost bag that contains all the necessary digestive enzymes and acids. Thus, cellular waste products, damaged cell parts, and spent protein molecules are chopped up, removed, and once again compounded to create new building materials and cell fuel.

That's also the reason why little muscle loss is experienced during times of fasting—provided the muscles continue to be trained and strengthened. This likely allowed our ancestors to survive even for long periods without food.

Galina Shatalova's Experiment[7]

Proof of the validity of this theory was provided by the Russian physician Galina Shatalova in the summer of 1990. She conducted a scientific experiment to discover whether it was possible for people who had survived severe diseases (diabetes, high blood pressure, pyelitis, liver cirrhosis, cancer) to be exposed to extremely high levels of physical and psychological stress. All of her study participants had been healed through caloric restriction and a balanced, plant-based diet.

All of the participants ate only four hundred calories a day, in the form of honey and raisins, and drank only half a liter of green tea, while walking up to twenty miles per day. And the results were amazing: The experiment was concluded earlier than expected, since the participants reached their goal in only sixteen days instead of twenty. And they felt great! They had retained their normal weight and even increased their muscle mass.

The conclusion we can draw from this is that autophagy released so many amino acids from the body's old proteins that the training regimen enabled participants not only to retain their muscle mass, but also to increase it.

The Miracle Molecule: Ketone

Ketone bodies (ketones, for short) are fatty acid molecules that develop when fat reserves are metabolized. In normal energy metabolism using glucose, the body needs large amounts of oxygen, which in turn produces many free oxygen radicals. Free radicals are destructive particles that can cause extreme damage to the cell walls as well as to genetic material.

Since energy production with ketones requires considerably less oxygen than energy production with glucose, this results in considerably fewer aggressive radicals. Fat breakdown begins as early as after twelve hours of fasting. Dangerous abdominal fat in particular (see pages 24 to 25) is converted to ketones. Ketones have always been the emergency source of energy in times of hunger; we know that they supply the heart, the brain, and all other vital organ systems with energy. They also activate the nerve cells and enable the production of new brain cells from brain stem cells.

Nature has wisely seen to it that neurotransmitters such as serotonin are created as needed. These reinforce any starvation period by maintaining high spirits. That may be the reason why I'm particularly efficient and creative during my daily fasting periods in the morning and early afternoon. It's also true that people who fast suffer less from neurological afflictions such as depression,[8] anxiety, Parkinson's disease,[9] and dementia.[10]

Ketones have the effect of soothing all chronic inflammatory processes (see page 21), such as those found in autoimmune diseases (allergies, Hashimoto's disease, multiple sclerosis, rheumatism) and in lifestyle diseases (high blood pressure, diabetes, heart attack, obesity). Fasting reduces pain, lowers blood pressure, and normalizes blood sugar values as well as reducing allergy symptoms. Ketones also decrease the level of LDL cholesterol ("bad" cholesterol) and thus contribute to better heart health—and they "starve" cancer cells in the truest sense of the word, since cancer cells are dependent on a certain level of blood sugar.

Carbs Are Essential

Genetically speaking, ketones are not designed to be the only sources of energy. There lies a major misunderstanding: If you stop eating carbs for a long period of time, as suggested by proponents of the keto diet, your metabolism will eventually shift to ketones. But that results in consequences that can be dangerous to human health. Why? Acidosis, one of the largest threats to our health, is massively fueled by the consumption of meat and other animal products. Even the brain is affected, since significantly reducing carbohydrate intake means providing the body with less sugar, which the body in turn has to generate by metabolizing it from amino acids and body fats, a difficult process.

Avoid Acidosis

People who eat mostly processed foods, meat, cold cuts, cheese, and other dairy products and get little exercise are "over-acidifying" their bodies, leading to acidosis. Since even very small deviations in the acid-base balance of our blood can be life-threatening, our body has developed emergency buffer systems: While the lungs take over short-term regulation by removing acids with the exhalation of carbon dioxide, the kidneys continually expel acids. Even our bones and fascia help to maintain a stable acid-base balance, for example, by releasing calcium when the blood becomes too acidic. Chronic acidosis, however, tends to withdraw too much calcium from the bones, resulting in osteoporosis.

Furthermore, chronic acidosis reduces the water-binding capacity of the connective tissue. Normally, the water contained in the joint cartilage is used as a buffer that can be pressed out like a sponge if need be. Once the stress is removed, the connective tissue reabsorbs the water. If too many acids settle between the cells and the connective tissue, the connective tissue loses the capacity to absorb water.

The results can be wide-ranging. The joints exhibit reduced mechanical buffering, and the connective tissue and fascia become less resilient, eventually turning stiff and inflexible. The risk of injury rises. The body tissues dry out and slowly become "polluted." The interstitial cell fluid cannot cope with the metabolic waste products emerging from the cells, and getting new supplies to the cells becomes more difficult. Signals can no longer be properly transmitted, paving the way for the development of severe diseases.

But physical activity, deep breathing, and an alkaline diet that includes lots of fruits and vegetables can reverse these processes. In the long term, it's best for your overall health if ketones are repeatedly created during intermittent fasting—just as nature intended. To that end, it is imperative that you consume *healthy* carbohydrates at your meals. This allows you to enjoy all the health benefits and get rid of superfluous fat without giving up carbs altogether.

Stopping the Growth of Cancer Cells

Valter Longo (see pages 13 to 14) was able to prove in animal experiments that the growth of cancer cells could be slowed using intermittent fasting—even in subjects that were already sick. In one study, the mice in the fasting group tended to live longer than those in the non-fasting groups. And the observation that the fasting mice suffered less from the aftereffects of chemotherapy and radiation therapy piqued the interest of the researchers.[11]

The initial studies done with patients revealed that the results from animal experiments could be replicated in humans: A study of thirty-four women with breast cancer or ovarian cancer at the Charité hospital in Berlin headed by Professor Andreas Michalsen confirmed the observations seen in mice: The women suffered from fewer negative aftereffects of chemotherapy, and their quality of life was higher than those in the control group that did not practice intermittent fasting.[12]

Initial Explanations

One explanation for this result could be that healthy cells go into "hibernation" during times of starvation, thus reacting exactly opposite to cancer cells, which get their "marching orders" from cancer growth genes, or oncogenes. Oncogenes program cancer cells to commence activity, to divide, multiply, and survive. Thus, the cancer cells do *not* adapt to the emergency situation the body is experiencing during chemotherapy or radiation therapy and just continue growing. So, while the healthy cells take cover, the cancer cells remain in action and are affected more intensely than the healthy cells by the therapy aimed at them.

The sugar deficit that occurs during fasting periods is another reason why cancer cells starve to death. To survive, most of them need "quick" simple sugars, such as white sugar, refined white flour, sweet drinks, chocolate, or other sweets. During the many hours of intermittent fasting, however, all the sugar drains from the blood so that the cancer cells receive no sustenance. And because no insulin is secreted in the absence of sugar, this also reduces the activity of the cancer cells, since insulin promotes cancer growth by boosting the synthesis of the growth factors.

No cancer can be completely healed through (intermittent) fasting alone. But regular, longer periods of food abstinence, combined with forgoing fast-release carbohydrates, can be especially helpful in supporting standard therapeutic approaches, like chemotherapy and radiation. In any case, cancer patients should discuss with their doctor before beginning any fasting regimen.

Antiaging Enzymes Take Off

Biologists and geneticists David A. Sinclair and Lenny Guarente, after researching the mechanisms of aging for two decades, made a groundbreaking finding: They discovered sirtuins, genes that can increase longevity.[13] Sinclair and Guarente determined that this particular family of enzymes has the ability to maintain the remediation and repair of the cells and their defenses, completely independent of age. The main task of the sirtuins is to enable the organism to survive, even under the harshest of circumstances, such as heat or lack of water or food.

Sirtuins are proteins that serve to protect the cells—they repair our DNA (which in turn contains the cells' genetic information). They protect our genome and ensure the lifetime of the cell. Every human being can profit from this mechanism by activating the sirtuins—through fasting—since sirtuins are activated only when the body assumes that nourishment is no longer forthcoming.

Activated Sirtuins = Long Life

For sirtuins to work properly, the stomach must be empty. As a result, the digestive coenzyme NAD (nicotinamide adenine dinucleotide) will have nothing to do, allowing it to become a supporter and activator of sirtuin molecules. The cellular repair work will commence immediately, mending the permanent damage caused by an unhealthy diet, negative environmental conditions, mental stress, and lack of physical exercise. This repair mechanism in the DNA of all individual cells explains why intermittent fasting allows us to live longer.

Sirtuins are the most well-known enzymes responsible for extending our lifetime. They are cell-protecting proteins—counterparts to free radicals. As long as they remain active, they are able to maintain or improve our state of health and effectively lengthen our life. Rather impressive!

Serotonin Release

In humans, the "happiness hormone" serotonin is responsible for our good moods, by biochemically activating certain parts of the brain. A number of things, however, can obstruct or even prevent these good feelings from occurring: an overly full stomach, aggravation, stress, strain, dissatisfaction. These negative conditions use up too much of our serotonin and cause us to seek out a compensatory means of satisfaction, often in the form of more food. Then, the next bad day is on the horizon. This vicious circle may even lead to depressive disorders, anxiety, and extreme loss of energy.

Intermittent Fasting Feels Good!

From the moment you decide to start intermittent fasting, you break through the gloominess. The "time-out" taken between meals regulates the body's hormonal balance and ensures that serotonin can work its wonders. That, too, can be explained by looking at our evolutionary development: During a famine, it was imperative that humans did not lose all hope for the future. In order to survive, they had to remain mentally strong and in relatively good spirits. Here again ketones play a decisive role, since they are responsible for increasing the amount of serotonin in the body. That's why intermittent fasting feels so good.

Inflammation in the Body

Inflammation is often misunderstood, as it is often considered to be something bad for you, something that has to be stopped. But inflammation can actually be a good thing, since it "ignites" a healing process the body needs to survive.

Chronic Inflammation
Chronic inflammation, on the other hand, is a genetically unforeseen process that occurs because repair activities were not properly concluded. Although it is a well-known medical fact that inflammation is supposed to maintain or reestablish

the integrity of the body, doctors often prescribe anti-inflammatory drugs to combat it. For example, inflammation of the Achilles tendon, which arises when the tension in the calf muscles becomes too great, leads to micro tears and swelling of the tendon: The body attempts to repair the damage, and pain ensues. If the tension on the muscles is not reduced, further tears occur, and the original inflammation becomes chronic, since the repair action cannot be completed. Instead of normalizing the muscular-fascial tension, the treatment is often to pump steroids into the tendon, abruptly ending the body's repair mechanism. So, it's no surprise that the tendon will never fully heal and may continue to tear.

Intermittent Fasting Puts an End to Inflammation

Inflammation stops naturally—and thus the body heals—only if it has been fully carried out. That means that the metabolic "accident" has been eliminated or the proper structure has been reinstated. The healthier we live, the quicker this process can take place. But if we try to put an end to inflammation with a medical Band-Aid, we effectively interrupt the body's natural healing process. Intermittent fasting supports the healing of inflammation by allowing the repair process to take its course. I have observed in many patients that their inflammation marker CRP (C-reactive protein) returns to normal upon practicing intermittent fasting.

Healthy Fasting Sleep

Humans sleep away about one third of their lifetime. And yet, as we sleep, our body is actually working in high gear. On average, we wake up around thirty times a night—we shift around and turn over many times to prevent circulatory problems and to regulate our body heat. Generally, however, we do not remember these waking phases, unless we stay awake for longer than three minutes. Waking up in the middle of the night is normal—these "sleep disturbances" are not the problem we often think they are. If you wake up in the middle of the night, you usually simply doze off again.

Hormones Regulate Our Sleep Patterns

The best way to obtain restful sleep is to maintain a properly functioning hormonal system. This helps to eliminate the "waste products" from the previous day and to provide the body with sufficient energy to get through the coming day. The body downregulates its temperature, which in turn activates the antiaging enzymes (see pages 20 to 21). In a well-organized process, the various hormones alternate

Intermittent Fasting and the Intestines

Are you familiar with the feeling you get in the pit of your stomach when you're excited? Or the bad feeling you get when you fail to listen to your gut instinct and make a bad decision?

THE SMALL INTESTINE

Our small intestine has as many nerve cells as our brain, including many cell types, signal substances, and receptors that are identical to those found in the brain. It produces over forty different psychoactive substances that influence our mental well-being. For example, 90 percent of the serotonin in our body is produced and stored in the lining of the intestine. Our moods are closely related to our digestive system, and thus our "intestinal brain" is the "overachiever" of our entire body. The small intestine also breaks down our food and plays a huge role in our immunity, which is why natural healing has long considered the intestine to be the seat of health.

THE MICROBIOME

The sheer number of bacteria present in our intestine—ten times that of the cells that make up our body—tells us something about the variety of the tasks this system has to conquer. This is the microbiome. The makeup of the colonies of bacteria that populate our intestine differs depending on our diet, our emotional state, and the state of our health in general. Generally, the greater the variety, the more effective our digestive system is at fulfilling its manifold duties.

SUPPORTING YOUR INTESTINAL MICROBIOTA

Fasting can support a healthy intestinal system. Our "good" intestinal bacteria are protected by certain ketones, beta-hydroxybutyrate acid, and the time-out period our intestine experiences during fasting. Otherwise, they are dominated and held in check by the "bad" intestinal bacteria. Fasting allows the good ones to gain the upper hand and to multiply. Fasting for sixteen hours a day is the best probiotic we could ever wish for to ensure the buildup of healthy intestinal microbes.

performing their respective duties: The sleep hormone melatonin ensures long phases of deep sleep; the most important sleep hormone, somatotropin (human growth hormone), allows children to grow and repairs the cells in adults, stimulating the creation of new cells and making us feel like we could "leap tall buildings" in the morning. The male sex hormone testosterone builds up muscle and breaks down fat. The hormone leptin dampens our hunger impulses at night and into the daytime. The thyroid gland is also active at night, producing hormones and preparing for the next day's important metabolic work. Beginning at about 3:00 AM, the stress hormone cortisol starts preparing the body for the wake-up phase.

Say Goodbye to Sleep Disorders

Sleep disorders can be tremendously damaging to quality of life. But they can be remedied. You do not need to resort to sleeping pills or go through special tests in sleep laboratories, since the main reason often lies in an overfull stomach. Eating a late evening meal, especially one difficult to digest, is a bad combination for good sleep and hinders the body from getting its much-needed nightly respite. Deep sleep phases are virtually impossible on a full stomach. The result is a feeling of leaden heaviness the next morning, making it difficult to get out of bed.

Many people think this is "normal," because it's what they're used to. But it doesn't have to be that way. Eat your final meal of the day, if possible, at about 6:00 PM (8:00 PM at the very latest). And make it a relatively light meal with few carbohydrates (see page 93). For your stomach to be more or less empty when you go to bed, we suggest taking a walk after the evening meal. You will find some wonderful recipes for evening meals in the 14-Day Program in this book (see pages 101 to 132) as well as in the recipe section for the third meal of the day (see pages 212 to 249).

Watch the Belly Fat Melt Away

As you already know, intermittent fasting speeds up fat burning. It's quite interesting: Ketones attack the unhealthy belly fat (visceral fat), which is responsible for cardiovascular problems, autoimmune diseases, and dementia, since it produces many more fat cell hormones than other fat cells, causing inflammation. This fat silently attaches itself to the organs in the abdominal cavity and remains invisible from the outside. Only when the body gains more weight overall does it come to be seen in the belly. The way your body fat is distributed makes a difference in your health: Belly fat (as seen in bodies with an "apple" shape) is unhealthier (leading to obesity-related ailments and diseases), as opposed to fat around the hips ("pear" shape).

Belly Fat Blinds Us from Feeling Full

Belly fat causes us to be voracious eaters, since it prevents leptin, the "I'm-full-now" hormone, from being recognized by the brain. Effectively, we then never feel full. It gives us the wrong impression that our body needs more food, leading to our regularly consuming too many calories. This is often coupled with insulin resistance and eventually the development of type 2 diabetes: the plague of many young people today. The disturbed sugar metabolism that ensues leads in turn to even higher blood lipid levels and dreaded cardiovascular diseases.

Belly Fat Leads to Inflammation

Belly fat causes cytokines to be emitted. These are neurotransmitters that cause inflammation and effectively trigger a chronic state of inflammation throughout the entire body. This in turn promotes vascular diseases, which eventually may lead to heart attack or stroke. Belly fat also produces the inhibitors that prevent blood clots from being dissolved. This fosters even larger blood clots (thromboses) that

WHO SHOULDN'T PRACTICE INTERMITTENT FASTING?

Children and adolescents should eat whenever they are hungry. And, as a rule, they naturally do just that. I would never force a child to eat something in the morning. What I would do, however, is make sure that the child gets healthy and delicious foods to eat at school, regardless of age. Further, people suffering from eating disorders of all types should be especially careful before embarking on an intermittent fasting diet. If you have an eating disorder, your goal should not be to lose weight with intermittent fasting—please consult your doctor before you start.

then either stick to the walls of the blood vessels or break free and cause embolism in the heart or the brain.

Fasting Increases Stem Cell Production

Valter Longo discovered that fasting causes a decrease in the number of white blood cells. During fasting, the body recycles old immune cells and, at the same time, activates the production of new ones with greater efficiency. Researchers used to think that these immune cells grew weaker over time, and that there was no way to influence this process. This is the idea behind the assumption that, as people grow older, they are generally more vulnerable to disease. Today, however, we know that regular fasting, and especially intermittent fasting, has the ability to "switch on" the regeneration button and to activate the signal paths for stem cells created by the circulatory and immune system. Furthermore, Valter Longo's research team determined that fasting lowers a particular enzyme called PKA (protein kinase A),[14] which improves the regulatory and self-renewal capacities of the body as well as its pluripotency (the ability of stem cells to differentiate into any of the body's three germ layers: endoderm, mesoderm, and ectoderm). All of these processes improve the health of the body and increase its lifetime. Stem cells can turn into any type of cell: organ lining, muscle, bone, blood, skin, nerves, and more. Thus, intermittent fasting is the key to remolding the physical body as well.

The Proof Is in the Eating

Modern medical research is very reticent about directly transferring the impressive results of intermittent fasting from animal experiments to humans. Long-term results are still being studied, and it is virtually impossible to have humans fast over long periods of time under laboratory conditions. And, of course, many other lifestyle parameters may influence the results. But don't let this scare you away from doing your own study—on yourself! Only then can you really know how intermittent fasting will affect you.

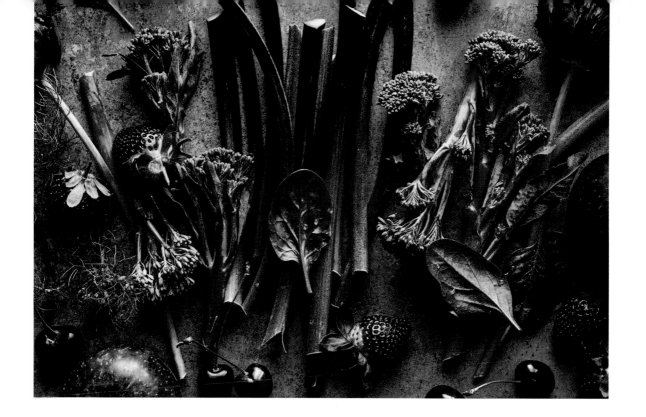

Intermittent Fasting as Therapy—from A to Z

Drugs are generally able to block or activate only a very limited part of our metabolism. Often, however, they dive deeper and disrupt complex processes, which in turn can produce strong side effects. As a doctor, of course, I won't avoid prescribing drugs in life-threatening situations. But I do prefer to apply them, if possible, concomitantly with other, more natural methods.

The Holistic Alternative

Fasting is the most important method we have at our disposal to enable the body to activate its genetically "built-in" powers of self-healing. My motto has always been: Everyone can understand how to stay healthy! We should not presume that you first have to understand the highly complicated biochemical and biophysical processes in order to know what you can do to promote your own health. This section is concerned with the most common diseases we experience. You'll learn why intermittent fasting functions as an important preventive measure for all of these diseases, and why you can expect improvement or even complete healing from intermittent fasting.

The Hormesis Principle

Any practitioner or proponent of natural medicine knows that short phases of stress can be beneficial to humans; these phases provide impulses for self-regulation, the activation of our natural, endogenic healing powers. This effect is known as the "hormesis principle" or "adaptive response," and has long been implemented in holistic therapeutic methods. It includes cold and warm stimuli (e.g., sauna, Kneipp cold water applications) as well as indulging in sea air or mountainous climates. Well into the last century, many sanatoriums were based on this principle.

Fever: Better than Medicine

Fever is also a natural stimulus function of the body. If you stop a fever with medicine, the symptoms may be soothed or eliminated, and the patient appears to get "better." It's tempting, but in the end, it's hardly a long-term solution, since it doesn't allow the body to conclude the "work" it should be doing to heal itself. Have you ever, upon feeling a cold coming on, swallowed a pill to reduce the fever and then gone to work? Don't do that! Suppressing these common ailments prevents the body from eliminating the source of the problem, and the immune system "unlearns" how to function properly. The body's "inner doctor" needs that stimulus to activate the immune system so that it can dispose of the pathogen on its own.

What Does All That Have to Do with Intermittent Fasting?

Research on fasting has discovered that a small stimulus, a slight surge of inflammation, occurs at the beginning of every fasting period. This upends our physiology and triggers whole chains of biochemical reactions. For a short period of time, it produces stress hormones—necessary to trigger the repair processes that are so essential to fasting. Valter Longo discovered that the stress comes first, followed by stem cell production.[15] If a disease has already started to emerge, our body is exposed to constant stress. But during fasting, our body will throw all its available means into activating the healing process. I've seen complete recovery in patients who begin to practice intermittent fasting.

Get Healthier

Whether it's used as a preventive method or to alleviate existing illnesses, intermittent fasting is the best way to care for your health. With intermittent fasting, your "inner doctor" takes over the therapy, and the inner doctor doesn't make mistakes. With diseases, intermittent fasting, together with a proper diet and exercise, is so powerful a method that often no other treatment is necessary. If the body cannot do the work on its own, this approach can be combined with other therapeutic methods. But my experience has taught me that this is rarely necessary.

Here's a short selection of the fantastic healing abilities of intermittent fasting, from A to Z. There's no disease that cannot be remedied with this trio—eat, fast, move—it gives your body the chance to heal itself.

A as in Acne

Acne is prevalent, especially among adolescents and younger adults. In times of stress associated with adolescence, dealing with blemished skin can be a major problem. Various salves and antibiotics often fail to work, since they do not actually attack the source. We should envision our skin as an extension of our small intestine. And if our intestine, like our brain, comes to be affected by a poor diet, it often shows up in our skin.

Causes

The growth hormone IGF-1 (see page 14) is instrumental in our body's growth processes. Too much food intake causes increased IGF-1 production. This is also true for products made from animal milk. The dermatologist and professor Bodo Melnik from the University of Osnabrück, one of the leading experts critical of the consumption of animal milk, proved that the additional rise in IGF-1 from the consumption of animal milk can lead to severe acne.[16]

How Intermittent Fasting Can Help

Intermittent fasting can influence the outbreak and spread of acne, sometimes even eliminating it completely. Fasting stops the excessive production of IGF-1 in the liver. Avoiding dairy products will have a similar effect, and avoiding dairy in conjunction with intermittent fasting is even better.

A as in Asthma

Asthma affects over three hundred million people worldwide[17]—someone dies from an asthma attack every three minutes. This is a result of allergens that can occur seasonally or sometimes year-round, such as dust, pollen, or animal hair. The allergies stemming from food do not get enough attention.

How Intermittent Fasting Can Help

I've observed that asthmatic symptoms decrease considerably with intermittent fasting, resulting in a reduced need for drug therapy. This is not surprising, considering the anti-inflammatory effects of intermittent fasting.

A study from 2007 revealed the positive effects of short-term fasting on overweight people suffering from asthma.[18] This study examined the lung function, general state of health, oxidative stress, and values of the highly sensitive inflammation gene CRP (see page 22). Fasting shows positive results as soon as after two weeks: Not only did the study participants lose 8 percent of their body weight, but their lung function also improved significantly, and their oxidative stress and inflammation markers were reduced. If you combine fasting with exercise and avoid all dairy products, asthma will often just disappear.

B as in Blood Pressure

Some 26 percent of people worldwide[19]—and 46 percent of Americans[20]—have high blood pressure (hypertension). But only half of them are even aware of it! And of the latter group, only 40 percent take medicine to control it. So, in the end only 25 percent see an improvement in their blood pressure values. Since increased blood pressure is one of the main risk factors for stroke, heart attack, and other cardiovascular diseases, you should determine whether your own blood pressure is too high. The optimal value for adults lies at about 120/80 (systolic/diastolic pressure).

If Your Blood Pressure Is Too High

If your blood pressure is too high, try to make some simple changes to your lifestyle to alleviate the situation. The American Heart Association suggests that patients first try to lower their blood pressure naturally, by changing their diet, engaging in physical activity, and managing stress levels.[21] These natural methods may be so successful that no drugs are necessary.

How Intermittent Fasting Can Help

I always recommend intermittent fasting as a means of lowering blood pressure. My experience has shown that it's often quite successful. If your blood pressure fails to go down fast enough, you can bridge any gaps with reduced doses of your usual antihypertensive drugs, and if intermittent fasting eventually does do the trick along with a proper diet and exercise, you may even be able to get off the drugs completely.

C as in Cancer

Up until now, fasting while suffering from cancer has been an absolute no-no. Unfortunately, many of my colleagues are still unaware of the recent research results on this topic. The reason is clear: Physicians are not required to attend any continuing education courses in nutrition. I myself obtained my knowledge through self-study, using my experience with my own patients.

The problem is that patients assume that their doctors have sufficient medical knowledge of proper nutrition. But instead of admitting to their own deficits, doctors will often tell their patients that it's best if they eat a balanced diet of whatever they find delicious.

Such statements make me sad and angry. Not only are patients, and here especially cancer patients, denied the wonderful healing powers of intermittent fasting, but it's also even described as "dangerous." Once you've read this book,

you will know more about the connection between intermittent fasting and health than most doctors do today. The effects I describe are unfortunately so little known to the public, even though Valter Longo confirmed the most striking ones long ago.

How Intermittent Fasting Can Help

Most cancer patients come to me for help after having gone through the conventional cancer treatments of chemotherapy and radiation. They then begin to combine these forms of treatment with my approach. I have found that intermittent fasting leads to a better ability to tolerate chemotherapy, with fewer side effects and better results (see page 19).

C as in Constipation

The most prevalent digestion problem in the Western world is constipation. In the United States alone, according to surveys, 16 percent of people suffer from constipation—and the real number is likely much higher. Most people take laxatives to solve the problem. But this doesn't actually address the cause of constipation—and it often makes it worse. Constipation is defined as irregular bowel movement primarily because of hardened stool, often in combination with considerable pain as well as bloating, abdominal cramps, and nausea. Normal stool frequency should be about two to three times a day, with a minimum of once a day. I do not condone the recommendation of at least three times a week; that, in my opinion, is already a sign of disturbed digestion and will be, in the long run, dangerous to your well-being.

Causes

Continual food intake causes an excessive load on our intestinal system, hampering digestion. Lack of exercise, too little fiber, and too many meat and dairy products in the diet as well as too few fluids, too many caffeinated drinks, and too much alcohol, further dehydrate the intestines and exacerbate the situation. The same is true for painkillers, blood pressure medicines, sedatives, antidepressants, cough suppressants, and iron supplements.

Healthy digestion is so important to our health, because one of the main causes of disease is the buildup of metabolic waste materials in our body. Constipation interferes with, or in some cases completely shuts down, many important metabolic processes. Cells can no longer be sufficiently supplied with oxygen and nutrients, and the body can no longer properly dispose of cellular waste. The cells die off, they degenerate, and the entire body becomes unbalanced. Suddenly, diseases break out or are simply attributed to age. A healthy digestive system is crucial for regularly eliminating excess matter from our bodies.

How Intermittent Fasting Can Help

A healthy intestinal system needs occasional time-outs as well as healthy, plant-based foods to develop good intestinal microbiota, which is largely responsible for keeping our immune system up and running. Regularly practicing physical exercises (see pages 62 to 87) does your digestion a big favor.

D as in Diabetes

Type 2 diabetes is reaching epidemic proportions all over the world. Nearly 9 percent of all Americans[22] are affected, though this number does not reflect those who have already developed insulin resistance, a precursor to diabetes, and a presumed large number of undiscovered cases.

Causes

The best treatment for diabetes is understanding how insulin secretion works in the circulatory system. The pancreas of a healthy person steadily secretes small quantities of insulin throughout the day, plus an increased amount after every meal. This hormone transports sugars to the cells to provide them with sufficient energy.

If we consume a diet mainly consisting of fruits and whole-grain products, which contain slow-release carbs, these will be steadily distributed at low-dose levels in the blood. The pancreas closely regulates the amount of insulin secreted. Fast-release carbs, on the other hand, namely, those found in sugary drinks, soft drinks, refined flour, chocolate, and sweets, quickly disperse in the blood stream and cause excessive insulin secretion.

If this continues over a longer period of time, the pancreas will eventually be overtaxed, and the cells will become insensitive to insulin due to the high secretion levels. This in turn triggers even greater insulin production, since the body always strives to supply the cells with enough sugar: A downward spiral begins. This new permanent high level of insulin then increases body weight, and insulin resistance gradually increases. This is considered the precursor to diabetes. If you already have diabetes and then adhere to the principles of the Paleo diet—something that is often recommended—this only worsens the disease! Too few of those afflicted know that fat and animal protein in particular are also responsible for the excess secretion of insulin. Even the fat hype so prevalent these days has a dark side to it: Type 2 diabetes reduces the amount of insulin produced so that the cells become resistant to sugar uptake.

Imagine insulin as a key that normally opens locks on the cells. In this case, it now no longer fits, because the lock has been glued shut by dietary fats, and the entire process comes to a halt. Now it makes no difference how much insulin is produced: The clogged-up cells can no longer absorb it. This mechanism may also be present in people without diabetes; even healthy people who consume a fatty meal may be limiting their body's capability to process it.

How Intermittent Fasting Can Help

Intermittent fasting together with a whole food, plant-based diet is the best therapy around for diabetes. The fasting period gives the pancreas the time-out it needs to regenerate. In the absence of insulin in the blood, fat can now be metabolized, ketones can be produced, and the negative effects of diabetes will start to disappear, piece by piece. The cells and the cell walls are freed of all the debris left behind. Healing can begin!

It has been my experience, again and again, that diabetics can embark on this path of healing. The success they experience day in and day out motivates even the most critical patient to stick to it. And what can be better for a diabetic than no longer having to give themselves insulin shots, and then hearing their doctor say the magic words: "You are healthy!"

F as in Fibromyalgia

Fibromyalgia is pain in the fibrous muscle tissue. Conventional medicine presently has no cure for it and only treats the symptoms. Generally, there's no sign of inflammation in the blood. The main symptom is pain in the soft tissue, including muscles, ligaments, connective tissue, tendons, and bursas. If a patient has a total of eight to twelve different pain points in their body, then the diagnostic assumption is one of fibromyalgia. Based on the typical symptoms, it is often considered a rheumatic disease. But some people also experience depressive moods, in addition to tiredness, sleep disorders, and stomach and intestinal disorders.

Causes

The symptoms are exacerbated by the weather, stress, poor diet, and lack of exercise. The most prevalent means of medical therapy are unsatisfactory, which isn't surprising: How do you treat something when you don't know the cause? Painkillers and antidepressants are the usual methods of choice, though they can have severe side effects. Yet they continue to be used, since there are no effective alternatives, and the goal is to relieve a patient's suffering. But my experience with pain therapy has shown that the cause of such pain is nearly always a combination of high tension in the muscles and fasciae, poor nutrition, mental stress, and environmental strain.

How Intermittent Fasting Can Help

Intermittent fasting and movement are the keys to relieving fibromyalgia: The exercises presented in this book normalize the tension in the motor system, and the healing effects of a plant-based diet serve to compensate for missing nutrients. Then, fasting can optimize the repair processes in the body such that the inflammation can heal, and a derailed metabolism can be made healthy again. Various dietary supplements can also contribute to the healing process.

H as in Heartburn

With heartburn (other terms include *pyrosis*, *acid reflux*, and *acid indigestion*), stomach acid flows upward into the esophagus. Typical symptoms range from pressure in the upper abdomen, a burning sensation in the throat, morning hoarseness, throat clearing, coughing, to a feeling of soreness behind the breastbone. If the inflammation is long term, it can result in chronic belching, difficulties swallowing, coughing, inflammation of the larynx, asthma, and, in the worst case, esophageal cancer. The usual cause of heartburn is the improper closing of the lower esophageal sphincter (the muscle that connects the esophagus to the stomach), which is supposed to function like a valve to prevent stomach acid from flowing backward and damaging the sensitive membrane of the esophagus.

Causes

One of the main reasons for heartburn is increased tension of the diaphragm and its fascia, caused largely by shallow breathing. Since the diaphragm surrounds the area around the esophageal sphincter, this increased tension interferes with the sphincter's function and allows stomach acid to flow back into the esophagus. Often, this is accompanied by a hiatal hernia, in which the upper stomach bulges through the diaphragm. But it is the disturbance of the sphincter that actually causes the heartburn. If, in addition, one eats heavy, fatty, or spicy meals, combined with alcohol, nicotine, or coffee, the pressure in the stomach increases and heartburn ensues. Stress can also exacerbate heartburn, since it increases the existing muscle tension.

How Intermittent Fasting Can Help

Intermittent fasting positively affects both the main cause as well as the various other triggers of heartburn. The physical exercises provided in this book can help to release the tension in the diaphragm. Daily

fasting also gives the stomach the time it needs to "tidy" things up and relaxes the entire intestinal system. People who tend to suffer heartburn at night should not eat at least four hours before going to bed. It's also recommended that heartburn sufferers cut down on their intake of sweets, fatty foods, animal products, and stimulants of all types.

H as in Heart Disease

Today, heart disease is the largest killer of people in Western countries, followed by cancer. Sudden death, heart attack, and stroke are the greatest dangers stemming from heart disease.

Causes

Heart disease generally occurs following arteriosclerosis, the thickening and hardening of the walls of the arteries, which is the result of modern lifestyle choices: poor diet and the absence of physical exercise. Disorders like high blood pressure and type 2 diabetes are nearly 100 percent self-induced. But all of the risk factors for heart disease (increased blood pressure, high blood sugar, excess body fat around the waist, and abnormal cholesterol levels—sometimes expressed with the term *metabolic syndrome*), can be reversed.

How Intermittent Fasting Can Help

I've been working with patients now for over thirty years and have seen many of them become healthy once again. That is why I encourage you to take the reins of your healing process in your own hands. Even arteriosclerosis can be reversed. After four to six weeks of my program, your blood values will change for the better, and symptoms like shortness of breath and angina pectoris will improve. After a year's time, your arteries will be like new.

M as in Migraine

Today, 12 percent of the American population—including children—suffer from migraines. It's the third most prevalent illness in the world.[23] But the exact reasons behind these headaches are often difficult to discern, when they're not caused by brain tumors or problems with the cervical vertebrae. So, instead of treating the unknown cause, the first line of attack is to prescribe painkillers that suppress the pain.

Causes

In my experience, frequent causes are extreme tension in the muscles and fasciae of the cervical vertebrae and head. This, in turn, causes tension in the neck, headaches, and migraines. The cause of the tension is often a lack of movement and long periods of sitting. But stress, improper diet, and any number of environmental factors can also increase this tension. Thus, we are dealing here with alarm signals that serve to prevent structural damage or excessive strain on the cervical vertebrae, particularly on the disks. If these alarms are ignored long enough or suppressed with painkillers, permanent damage may ensue, which is exactly what the body was trying to warn us about: slipped or herniated disks or disk protrusions, facet joint arthrosis, or spondylolisthesis.

How Intermittent Fasting Can Help

By practicing intermittent fasting in conjunction with physical exercises, you can avoid many of the causes associated with migraine. The exercises in particular will lengthen muscles and fasciae in the neck and head. A plant-based diet, combined with the effects of fasting, can be instrumental in normalizing the tension in muscles and fasciae. This, I've found, makes migraine headaches curable.

N as in Neurological Diseases

Neurological diseases include depression, anxiety, concentration disorders, dementia, Parkinson's disease, and multiple sclerosis, to name just a few.

Causes

Our modern lifestyle has led people to turn to the keto diet to gain energy. But the ketones are what have such a fantastic effect on our neurological system. For example, for many years now, fasting has been known to tackle epilepsy.

How Intermittent Fasting Can Help

Fasting as therapy has been used in Russia for many decades as a solution for mental disorders, such as schizophrenia.[24]

Mark Mattson, renowned Johns Hopkins neurobiologist, proved in animal experiments that the fasting brain produces endogenous opiates.[25] Further, the nerve growth factor BDNF (brain-derived neurotrophic factor) increases considerably during fasting (and after exercise). This factor is responsible for proper brain function, keeping our brain healthy and us in good spirits.

Another important task, once again, is played by the ketones, which provide the energy for our brain during fasting (see pages 17 to 19). Overall, they have a healing effect on neurological and mental disorders. Even the inevitable course of congenital neurological disorders seems to be delayed by fasting.[26]

O as in Overweight

Worldwide obesity has nearly tripled since 1975—39 percent of adults aged eighteen years and over are now overweight.[27] But obesity is a preventable condition, and the main cause lies in the excessive consumption of animal products (meat, dairy) and sugary foods. Simply put, we eat too much food—and too much unhealthy food at that.

Causes

The hormone leptin regulates our energy balance and our weight. We produce leptin in our fatty tissues. The more these tissues are filled, the more leptin is secreted and flows into our bloodstream. Our brain registers this increase in leptin, giving us the feeling of satiety; we feel happy, full, and satisfied. When we fast, on the other hand, leptin is not present in our blood: Our brain sends out an alarm signal, telling us we're hungry. If we ignore that signal and don't eat anything, it then activates our evolutionary survival mode.

But why do people who are overweight, with full fat deposits and high leptin levels, still have an insatiable hunger? A few years ago, researchers discovered that an extremely high level of insulin masks leptin in the bloodstream: The brain thinks—wrongly—that the body is still in a state of famine.[28] The main culprits here are processed sugar, sweets, sugary soft drinks, fast food, and processed foods. Other consequences of a chronically high level of insulin are a fatty liver, insulin resistance, and type 2 diabetes.

How Intermittent Fasting Can Help

Intermittent fasting lowers insulin levels, making leptin visible once again to the brain. Whether the reason behind your excess weight lies in an underactive thyroid gland, in your hormones, in depression, or because of a genetic disposition, intermittent fasting will enable you to reach your ideal weight! Week after week it ensures that fat is burned and turned into ketones (see pages 17 to 19). Your mood lightens, your disease symptoms disappear, your lipid fat values improve, and your other blood values return to their normal level. You become more agile, happier, and stronger, day after day. All this despite eating two to three meals a day!

P as in Pain

In my experience as a pain specialist, I have observed that patients who optimize their diet are better able to control—and sometimes eliminate—their back pains or migraine headaches. Yet, like many other therapists, I did not, at first, understand the cause of these successes.

Causes

Today, we know how this works: Generally speaking, when muscular-fascial tension is too high, pain ensues—this is true for nearly every single pain situation we know of. Pain in our musculoskeletal system often occurs in the absence of crucial nutrients, like vitamins B, D, and E, so special dietary supplements can help to alleviate these deficits.

How Intermittent Fasting Can Help

Our bodies react to positive stimuli by relaxing; the intermittent fasting program introduced in this book can help to relieve most pain conditions. Intermittent fasting decreases inflammation and therefore can reduce pain for example for patients with inflammatory arthritis.[29] Pain therapy can also help to "turn off" this high tension level, and proper execution of the exercises in this book (see pages 62 to 87) can help to alleviate pain. I recommend intermittent fasting particularly for patients suffering from severe chronic pain, such as that associated with fibromyalgia and multiple sclerosis.

R as in Rheumatism

Rheumatism is a series of autoimmune diseases caused by chronic inflammation in the body.

Causes

We know without a doubt that animal products, such as meat, eggs, fish, and dairy, promote or even cause inflammatory processes in our body. Add chronic stress and sleep deprivation to the equation, and our immune system becomes overtaxed. It can no longer differentiate between good and bad and ends up attacking itself.

How Intermittent Fasting Can Help

Once our immune system has "gone haywire," it needs a lot of support and considerable time to be brought to its "senses" once again. But that's exactly what intermittent fasting can do. It's almost like pressing the "reset" key on a computer—it reboots and reorganizes the body, in order to restart our immune system's healing and repair program. It's well known that fasting can help people with rheumatism. But not all of these research results have reached the rheumatologists, an unbelievable state of affairs if you remember that this particular autoimmune disease, with its nearly unbearable pain, is a prime example of how intermittent fasting can bring relief in only a short time.[30]

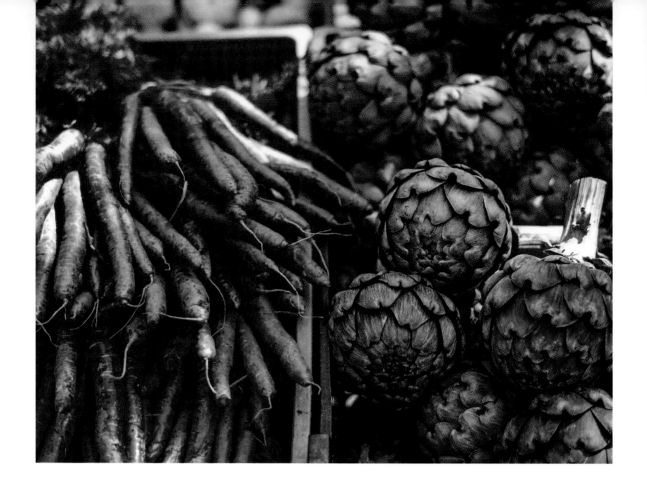

Formula for a Healthy Life: Vegan Fasting

Why is it better to eliminate animal products? What does our body need to stay healthy and fit? What ingredients are toxic—and why? Here, you'll find all the answers to your questions.

Plant-Based vs. Animal-Based Foods

Modern scientists are convinced that our ancestors subsisted largely on a plant-based diet. But over the course of our evolutionary history, humans have never been completely vegan: We have always been dependent on animal foods as well—for our survival, but also for cultural, economic, and social reasons.

Today, however, meat and dairy products are no longer luxury goods, and most societies, at least in industrialized nations, can afford to eat a high-quality and exclusively plant-based diet. There is an ample supply of plant-based foods available, enough to meet our daily nutritional requirements.

We should all strive to eat this "new" type of diet, since the facts are clear: A plant-based diet promotes health and prolongs life. For example, a study at Harvard University showed that a diet that replaced red meat with healthy plant proteins reduced the risk factors for cardiovascular incidents as well as overall mortality.[31]

If, however, you prefer not to remove meat and animal products from your diet entirely, it's still possible for you to undertake a fasting diet. Just remember that the dose makes the poison: No more than 5 percent of your diet should consist of animal products! I wholeheartedly recommend a diet low in animal products—but I would be the last person to try to force you to give them up. Maybe you'll eventually decide to eat fewer meat and milk products, or you'll alternate

eating meat every other week. That works, too. Maybe you need to approach veganism slowly and carefully. You may want to start by eliminating eggs from your diet. Eggs can be full of pesticides, as the 2017 fipronil scandal demonstrated,[32] and studies have shown that eggs may increase risk of prostate cancer.[33]

Many of my patients start off by eliminating dairy products and processed meats from their diet, preferring fewer, higher-quality cuts of meat. Everyone can decide for themselves what is best for them. But I know this to be true: Every little bit of animal protein and fat you cut from your diet helps to make you healthier. And, over time, I'm convinced you'll notice that phasing out animal products has improved your quality of life—and you'll never turn back.

Buy Local and Sustainable

We all live lives that are a far cry from creating a sustainable and healthy world. But now's the time to finally do something about it! The first step could be buying more local and seasonal products, ideally from a local farmers market or from a supermarket that operates without plastic and without producing packaging waste.

Support your local organic farmers by eating seasonal fruits and vegetables. Try to purchase produce grown with no pesticides or herbicides. If everyone were to eat more consciously and conscientiously, with mostly local foods, it would make a huge difference in stopping environmental damage to our beautiful world. We can all do our part to make this world a better place—every little bit helps.

This task may be easier or harder, depending on where you live. It's likely going to be easier during the summer months when a broader selection of vegetables is available. Look at a seasonal growing calendar for your area to see what will be offered at your local farmers market or supermarket. The winter months can sometimes have fewer alternatives, but you can spice up your local offerings with organic foods from other regions of the country or the world, where certain fruits and vegetables are readily available even in December and January. When shopping, pay special attention to the ripeness of the fruits and vegetables and note where they come from. If only we would all become a little more adept at buying locally, it would profit both our health and the local (organic) agriculture. A final tip: If you feel the need to buy fewer avocados (as they may not be local to your area), substitute them with nuts, which contain many valuable fatty acids.

SHOULD WE BE EATING ANIMALS?

Whether we should eat animals is both a philosophical and an ethical question.

Many people like the taste of meat and are convinced that animal foods should be part of their diet; they think that animals exist to be eaten. Although I know that not all of my readers are fans of the vegan lifestyle, I would like to challenge that approach.

Would you eat your dog, your cat, or your beloved horse? You have a close relationship with your pets; they're your companions. So, do we eat cows, pigs, and sheep only because we don't have these same relationships?

Why Certified Organic Products?

Organic is better than conventional, hands down. A study at Newcastle University is presently the most comprehensive study on this matter. Headed by Marcin Baranski, this study reviewed a total of

343 publications from renowned journals dealing with the health ramifications of vitamins, secondary phytochemicals, antioxidants, chemical pesticides, nitrites and nitrates, and poisonous heavy metals such as cadmium, arsenic, and lead. The results were unambiguous: Organic crops have higher antioxidant activity and contain between 18 percent and 69 percent higher concentrations of antioxidants than conventional products.[34] These substances have been shown to prevent cancer, cardiovascular diseases, and neurodegenerative diseases. The study also showed that organic fruits contain more vitamin C and carotenoids than their conventional counterparts. Whereas organically grown plants have to defend themselves against negative environmental conditions, pests, and other stressors by creating their own antioxidants as a first line of defense, conventionally grown fruits and vegetables become "sluggish" and "lazy" when treated with pesticides. As a result, they cease producing their own health-promoting substances.

The study also uncovered the negative effects of pesticides and heavy metals. Organic fruits, for example, contained up to 48 percent less of the toxic metal cadmium than their conventional counterparts. Conventional crops were four times more likely to contain detectable pesticide residues. From this, it's clear that foods that are grown under natural environmental conditions are the healthiest for our bodies. This makes sense, if you recall that our genes cannot recognize these artificial substances and poisons that have been used in agriculture for only a few decades.

Fiber, Fiber, So Much Fiber

Fiber is found exclusively in plants. The main sources are legumes, whole grains, leafy greens, vegetables of all types, fruits, and nuts. The recipes found in this book are chock-full of these delicious and filling foods.

One of the main effects of dietary fiber is its ability to absorb fluids and swell up. This causes us to feel full earlier; roughage increases the overall volume of our stool and thereby prevents constipation. Any excess cholesterol attaches to the fiber and is excreted.

Diseases of the intestinal tract are on the rise, from food intolerance to chronic intestinal inflammation (ulcerative colitis, Crohn's disease) and colon cancer. There is reason to suspect that the level of fiber in modern diets lies well below that of our ancestors. The National Academy of Medicine recommends 38 grams of fiber per day for men under fifty years of age and 25 grams for women, and 30 grams for men and 21 grams for women over fifty years of age.[35] But I believe these recommendations are much too low: Our ancestors likely ingested more than twice that much. And these recommendations aren't always met. Fiber is of paramount importance to our entire digestive system, as it is responsible for establishing the proper climate for "good" bacteria to grow in our intestines. They in turn strengthen our immune system, 80 percent of which is located in our digestive system.

Vitamin B_{12}: A Crucial Ingredient for Vegans

Vitamin B_{12} can be found in animal products (eggs, meat, milk) as well as possibly in algae such as chlorella and nori. Vitamin B_{12} is responsible, among other things, for producing red blood cells, protecting our genes, stabilizing our nerves, and preventing cardiovascular diseases and cancer. If you do decide to take up a completely plant-based diet, you will need to supplement it with additional vitamin B_{12}. Since human beings have never been completely herbivorous throughout our evolutionary history, vitamin B_{12} deficiency was never a problem for our ancestors, since even small amounts of animal products suffice to satisfy our needs. But that's also a hint that humans have never consumed large amounts of animal products. Bacteria that naturally live in fruits and vegetables also produce this vitamin, so when we clean our fresh foods too thoroughly, we are also washing away the "good" bacteria and with them the vitamin B_{12}.

Vitamin B_{12} deficiency varies by age, affecting at least 3 percent of Americans aged twenty to thirty-nine years old, 4 percent of those aged forty to fifty-nine years, and 6 percent of those aged sixty years or over.[36] It should also be noted that 15 percent of people under sixty and 20 percent of those over sixty years of age were found to have a marginal depletion of vitamin B_{12} in their diet, despite consumption of animal products.[37] The reason lies in part in prescription drugs, which can hinder the stomach lining from properly absorbing vitamin B_{12}. Thus, a lack of vitamin B_{12} is not a problem exclusive to vegans, who generally are aware of the necessity to supplement their vitamin B_{12} intake. Omnivores are less likely to be aware of this and thus may suffer from a vitamin B_{12} deficit, affecting both their health and quality of life considerably.

The Truth About Protein

Protein is generally thought of as something derived from animal products—meat, fish, eggs, milk. Unfortunately, slogans such as "Got milk?" (created by the

California Milk Processor Board) have been burned into our brains. That might also be the reason why low-carb and Paleo diets—which are merely new versions of the controversial Atkins diet—are now making a comeback.

The Atkins Diet

The nearly complete renunciation of carbohydrates and the increase in consumption of fat and protein—that is the Atkins diet, which its founder said leads the body to burn fat and create ketones for energy generation (see pages 17 to 19). But the Atkins diet remains very controversial—in the short term, dieters often lose weight, but numerous studies have shown that this diet is unlikely to result in significant long-term weight loss and may actually lead to serious health problems.[38]

Problematic Animal Protein

It has often been said that a plant-based diet cannot provide a sufficient amount of protein. In fact, the opposite is true! What often makes us ill is the excessive consumption of animal-based protein. Professor Lothar Wendt, at the University of Frankfurt, was the first to discover this in the 1950s. He proved the existence of the protein storage disease thesaurismosis, in which the cell membranes literally become clogged up with too much animal

protein and are impermeable.

The World Health Organization (WHO) has classified processed meat products such as cold cuts, and possibly the meat of cows, pigs, sheep, and goats, as carcinogens.[39] According to a 2017 report by the American Institute for Cancer Research and the World Cancer Research Fund, daily intake of just 50 grams of processed meat products (the equivalent of one hot dog or a few strips of bacon) increases the risk of contracting colorectal cancer by 16 percent.[40] This information is shocking, especially if we consider that, for the year 2019, average meat consumption per capita was 223 pounds (101 kg). In 2009, a study by the American National Cancer Institute came to similar conclusions: A study of over five hundred thousand participants revealed that those with a high animal protein diet have a 25 percent higher risk of colorectal cancer, a 20 percent higher risk of lung cancer, and an up to 60 percent higher risk for esophageal and liver cancer. They also observed a connection with pancreatic cancer.[41]

The Issue with Milk

Professor Bodo Melnik's work demonstrates that milk isn't just a food—his study found that it's likely a "genetic transfection system," in which foreign DNA is introduced to the body's cells, stimulating postnatal growth.[42] Cow's milk activates the enzyme complex mTORC1 in the cells of the milk's intended recipient—the calf—activating cell division. Of special importance to mTORC1 activation are the essential amino acids that are highly concentrated in milk protein; they can lead to the additional secretion of other growth hormones such as insulin and IGF-1. Melnick's study stated that, like cow's milk for calves, human breast milk is the ideal food for infants, but persistent cow's milk consumption through adolescence and adulthood may lead to mTORC1-driven lifestyle diseases.[43]

Milk is not only a source of nutrition—it also contains signaling molecules that regulate further development through the transfer of genetic material in micro-ribonucleic acids (microRNAs).[44] MicroRNA regulates gene expression in all mammals; it turns off any "obstructive" protein molecules, which in turn leads to further and faster cell growth. In the growth period immediately after birth, these growth accelerators are necessary.

But when microRNA from cow's milk continues to enter the adult human body, it can lead to diseases such as obesity[45] (excessive stimulation of fat cells), diabetes[46] (overactivation of the insulin-producing islet cells of the pancreas), cancer[47] (increased mTORC1-dependent growth of cancer cells), dementia[48] (increased activation of protein biosynthesis in the nerve cells), acne[49] (overstimulation of the oil glands in the skin), and overall mortality.[50] If all of this is news to you, and you suffer from any of these ailments, you may want to consider giving up milk and milk products.

Plant-Based Protein Sources

There are many excellent sources of plant-based protein, such as legumes, fermented soy products (miso, natto, tempeh, tofu), beans, lentils, and peas. Nuts and seeds of all types (walnut, cashew, hazelnut, almond, hemp, chia) and whole grains such as quinoa, rice, buckwheat, corn, oat, millet, rye, and spelt are high-quality sources of protein.

Plants can provide our bodies with protein, without the massive negative side effects of animal products. Also, don't forget that meat, fish, eggs, milk, and their derivatives contain by-products of modern factory farming, such as antibiotics, insecticides, heavy metals, and hormones. That's what meat eaters are putting into their bodies! The reality of consuming animal products in today's world means it's ultimately healthier to reduce or eliminate animal protein altogether.

Carbohydrates: Yes!
Sugar: No!

Simple sugar is unhealthy. Carbohydrates that come from whole foods such as grains, seeds, legumes, vegetables, and fruits, on the other hand, are not just healthy but in fact necessary for our continued health. Unfortunately, the low-carb movement has created a lot of consumer uncertainty.

Our cells need glucose for energy, most importantly our brain and nerve cells and our red blood cells. To this end, our body stores sugar in the form of glycogen; these stores can cover all our energy needs for up to twenty-four hours. In addition to fats, carbohydrates are the most important energy sources we have to cover our daily needs: 1 gram of carbohydrates has four calories; 1 gram of fat has nine. We need these macromolecules to properly regulate our protein and fat metabolism.

We need these complex carbs, but we don't need sugar. The average American eats 42.5 teaspoons of sugar per day, way more than the recommended 13.3 teaspoons per day,[51] and excessive sugar consumption is responsible for many diseases. The simultaneous consumption of sugar and fat can cause catastrophic damage, leading to hyperphagia (abnormally increased appetite). Sugar is added to nearly every type of processed food—lurking in places you'd never expect.

The Difference Between Good and Bad Sugars

There are different types of sugar: simple sugars (monosaccharides), double sugars (disaccharides), and complex sugars. The most common simple sugars are glucose and fructose. Fruits contain fructose, but because of the accompanying amount of fiber and the many nutrients in fruit, the fructose does not cause the blood sugar level to increase quite as much. The double sugars include table sugar (sucrose) as well as malt sugar (maltose) and milk sugar (lactose); these are found largely in sweets, soft drinks, ice cream, and chocolate. They are dangerous because they do nothing but transport calories, and are responsible for quick increases in blood sugar levels.

Complex sugars are in fact complex carbohydrates made up of long sugar molecule chains. The most important type of complex sugar is starch, which is present in grains, potatoes, and legumes. Complex sugars increase the blood sugar level very slowly. The long sugar chains are gradually broken down before being absorbed in the bloodstream, allowing the blood sugar level to rise more slowly and the pancreas to produce insulin at a leisurely pace. And, as we all know by now, too much insulin will cause weight gain and illness.

The Fructose Trap

Fruit sugar, fructose, sounds like it should be healthy. But what's the real story here—and why is it responsible for so many more diseases? Many think that fruit sugar—because of its name—only exists in fruit. But it's worth noting that table sugar, whether white or brown, consists of a mixture of fructose and glucose. These two sugars are utilized differently by our body. Glucose is transported to the cells by insulin and directly turned

Prevent and Reverse Heart Disease

That's the title of a book by Caldwell B. Esselstyn, the doctor who turned Bill Clinton into one of the best-known vegans in the world. The former president was able to reverse the effects of his heart disease by adopting a vegan diet.

In 1985, Esselstyn initiated a strictly vegan diet among twenty-four patients with advanced coronary heart disease. Many of them had already had bypass operations. Six of the participants gave up after a few weeks, and their heart disease kept advancing. The remaining eighteen patients who stuck to the diet stayed healthy. The blood supply to their hearts improved, since their blood vessels were measurably larger.

THE ROLE OF ARGININE

A vegan diet triggers the inner layer of blood vessels to produce nitric oxide, one component of which is the amino acid arginine, which occurs naturally in legumes.[52] This substance prevents plaques from building up and helps to remove existing plaque.[53]

into energy on the spot. Any excess of glucose is stored as fat, leading to excess weight. Fructose was long thought to be "harmless" and was recommended to diabetics as a sugar replacement, since it does not lead to an immediate increase in blood sugar level. Fructose is transformed into glucose, energy, or fatty acids only in the liver, where insulin is not necessary. However, if too much fructose is ingested, it is turned into fat, leading to fatty liver disease—which affects about one hundred million Americans,[54] most of whom are not even aware of the problem, since they do not experience pain in the liver. As a result, the liver can no longer sufficiently

In 1998, three American scientists were awarded the Nobel Prize in Medicine for discovering how production of nitric oxide can affect the body. Nitric oxide in the body is responsible for widening blood vessels, helping to regulate blood pressure, initiating erections, battling infections, preventing formation of blood clots, and acting as a signal molecule in the nervous system.[55] Protein from animal sources, on the other hand, forms ADMA (asymmetric dimethylarginine), which displaces arginine, inhibiting nitric oxide production and increasing risk of cardiovascular disease.[56]

PREVENTING ARTERIOSCLEROSIS

Increased cholesterol in the bloodstream leads to the development of arteriosclerosis. If the level is too high, white blood cells try to remove the cholesterol from the blood, become overloaded, turn into foam cells, and burst, depositing this cholesterol into the cell walls. These deposits lead to inflammation of the cell walls and constriction of the blood vessels.

These high levels of cholesterol in the body can only stem from a diet heavy in animal products. With a completely plant-based diet, high levels of "bad" LDL cholesterol often disappear within a few weeks,[57] allowing the "good" HDL cholesterol to run its course.

detoxify the body, and patients suffer from a lack of energy. It can also lead to insulin resistance, the precursor to type 2 diabetes (see pages 32 to 34).

The Truth About Fat

Americans get about 35 percent of their nutritional energy from fats—firmly at the higher end of the recommended guidelines of 20 to 35 percent.[58] Most of this fat comes from animal sources: meats, eggs, and dairy products. And most of it is saturated fat, which is responsible for the development of inflammation in the body.[59] This has led to an increase in modern lifestyle diseases like obesity,[60] diabetes,[61] lipid metabolism disorders,[62] gout,[63] and cardiovascular diseases,[64] including high blood pressure, coronary artery spasm, stroke, and heart attack. Increased fat intake is also associated with allergies,[65] autoimmune diseases,[66] neurodegenerative diseases such as multiple sclerosis[67] and dementia,[68] and cancers of the intestine,[69] breast,[70] and prostate.[71] Animal foods also have a higher ratio of omega-6 fatty acids to omega-3 fatty acids than most plant-based foods. This excess of omega-6 fatty acids is another factor in the development of chronic inflammation.

Even a moderate reduction (20 to 30 percent) in the consumption of animal products can help to prevent diseases stemming from inflammation. The simplest way is to reduce the proportion of animal foods in your diet and use less fat and oil in preparing your meals (see more about trans fats on page 51).

Lower Your Cholesterol

The body produces its own supply of cholesterol, so there's no need to add extra cholesterol to our diet. In limited amounts, it serves as a building block for our hormones and cell membranes and is responsible for transporting fat-soluble vitamins in the bloodstream.

We can't live without cholesterol. It is present in all human cells and is an indispensable resource. For example, when exposed to sunlight, our body creates vitamin D from its own reservoir of cholesterol. The production of hormones such as estrogen, progesterone, and testosterone would not be possible without cholesterol.

High Cholesterol Is Not Inherited

There are some exceptional cases of inherited disorders of fat metabolism, but in my experience, these are very rare. When patients tell me their high cholesterol is genetic, since their father, grandfather, or uncle had it, the first question I ask them is about their own dietary behavior. It turns out that it is generally no different from that of my other patients with high cholesterol, which makes it clear that genes are not responsible.

What to Avoid

Artificial Additives

Additives are an integral part of our modern food industry. Food dyes, preservatives, and sugar substitutes and sweeteners have become big business ventures. Generally, they are artificially created and do not naturally occur in foods. Nearly all prepackaged food contains additives to maintain shelf stable quality. The US Food and Drug Administration (FDA) maintains a list of hundreds of approved additives that are deemed safe for us to ingest on a daily basis.[72]

But what most people don't know is that these lists change all the time, and the research findings are often contradictory. Additives once considered safe for consumption can easily be removed from these lists if negative effects are discovered. It's alarming that there have been no studies on the long-term or combined effects of these additives. The bottom line is that the healthiest foods are ones that occur naturally—plant-based whole foods with nothing artificial.

Trans Fats

Trans fats, which occur naturally in small quantities in meat and dairy products, are also created artificially in an industrial process that adds hydrogen to liquid vegetable oils to make them more solid. Since 2013, the FDA has determined that these artificial trans fats are not safe for human consumption.[73] The extreme temperatures used in heating and frying foods over a longer period of time changes the fat molecules and makes them extremely dangerous to human health. Imagine trans fats as a sticky mass that attaches to the walls of cells, blood vessels, and nerves, wreaking havoc on their functions.

Consumption of trans fats increases the risk of developing many modern illnesses such as cardiovascular disease, stroke, and type 2 diabetes.[74] They are found in french fries; potato chips; fried foods of all kinds; doughnuts, pastries, and other baked goods; spreads; breading; ice cream; processed meats; and even in granola bars and breakfast cereals.

At the store, pay attention to the ingredients on the labels. For example, you may find the words *(partially) hydrogenated oils*. These are trans fats. If possible, try to avoid these products. In unpackaged foods, however, it may be difficult to determine whether they contain trans fats.

AGEs: Less Well Known, but Just as Dangerous

AGEs (advanced glycation end products) are toxins that cause inflammation in the body, contribute to the aging process, and likely play a major role in the development of many diseases such as cardiovascular disease, atherosclerosis, kidney disease, and diabetes.[75] AGEs have a destructive effect on the brain and its cognitive abilities and promote neurodegenerative diseases such as dementia and Parkinson's disease.[76]

The largest dose of harmful AGEs enters the body when we eat heated, fried, grilled, dried, or smoked fats, proteins, and sugars. To date, some five hundred different foods have been tested for their AGE content. Meat (especially red meat), certain cheeses, fried eggs, mayonnaise, margarine, oils, and nuts have the highest levels of AGEs,[77] whereas plant-based foods have the lowest. How food is prepared plays a major role: Steaming or stewing produces much fewer AGEs than methods that expose the food to dry heat, such as frying, baking, and grilling. It's important to note that cigarette smoke also contains high levels of AGE.[78]

Gluten

Some ten thousand years ago, *Homo sapiens* began to cultivate twenty-five thousand different types of wheat from wild grasses. They continued to breed hybrids from wild einkorn wheat, creating what would become our common wheat, which was easier to process.

Modern high-performance wheat has little to do with ancient einkorn. In 1970, Dr. Norman Borlaug received the Nobel Peace Prize for his work on the development of genetically modified durum wheat. An implanted dwarf gene shortened the length of the wheat stalk and made the ears so much more profitable that India was able to increase its wheat crop three times over within ten years. After four years of growing this wheat, Mexico no longer needed to import it. The other side of the coin, however, is that these genetic modifications changed both the gluten genes and the gluten content considerably. This move may be responsible for the major increase in intolerance toward gluten: Between 1950 and 2005, the number of people suffering from celiac disease increased fivefold.[79]

Other grains contain gluten in its original form, such as rye, spelt, kamut, and barley. My patients have told me again and again that they have no problems at all with these grains but do suffer symptoms of gluten intolerance when they eat modern wheat. The typical symptoms are fatigue, distension, diarrhea, headache, poor concentration, and a ravenous appetite.

It is not my goal here to jump on the train of damning gluten. But I do suggest to my patients that they closely observe their habits if they suspect they are gluten intolerant. They should then avoid all gluten-containing grains for a period of four weeks, replacing them with gluten-free grains, legumes, and seeds. They should also be careful with processed foods that contain emulsifiers and stabilizers, which may contain gluten. If they notice a considerable improvement, then they know that they are indeed affected; if there is no change to their condition, they can and should continue to eat gluten-containing grains.

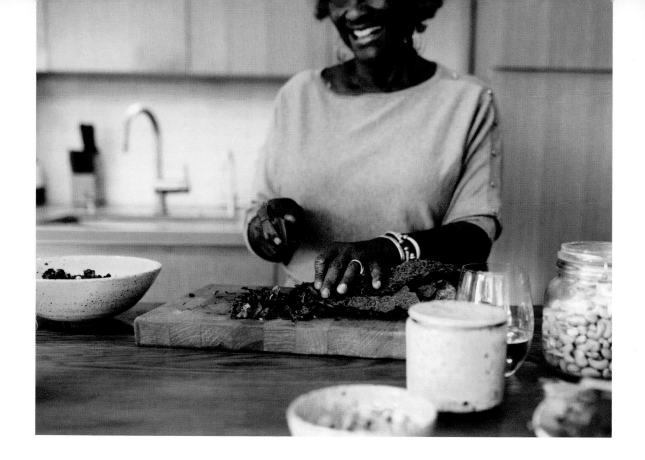

The 16:8 Rule

The idea behind intermittent fasting is simple: You have a window of eight hours a day in which you can eat. During this time frame, you eat two to three normal meals (all vegan, if possible), and then you fast for the following sixteen hours. The ideal eating time is between noon and 8:00 PM. This time span has proved advantageous, mainly because it's easiest for most people to adhere to. That's not surprising if you recall that we spend a large part of each day sleeping, when we don't eat anyway. So, if you, for example, eat your last meal at 7:00 PM and fast until the next day at 11:00 AM, you've made it! Now that wasn't so difficult, was it?

If, for some reason, you're unable to keep to these times (for example, when you're invited for a late dinner somewhere), just push the first meal of the next day back accordingly. If you want to eat breakfast early, move the last meal of the previous day up to an earlier time. The most important thing about intermittent fasting is that there should always be at least a sixteen-hour pause in your meals. Everything else is negotiable.

Long Fasts, Major Effect

The 16:8 rule is optimal for getting in the groove with intermittent fasting. Three meals a day are also optimal. Believe me, you won't ever go hungry.

Once you've determined how this new eating rhythm fits your needs, try eating just two meals a day and lengthening the intermittent fasting schedule to 18:6. That is, you eat all your meals within a six-hour window and fast for the remaining eighteen hours.

The rule is: The longer the fasting time, the more your body profits from the autophagy process (see page 16). It has more time to repair and recycle, more time to regenerate. This also means more time to break down body fat, especially dangerous visceral belly fat.

Some people prefer to eat only once a day. I have practiced this myself, for example, when I have to concentrate all day long on my work and don't want to be hit with the energy low that often occurs after a meal. On these days, I really look forward to that one meal. When 6:00 PM comes around, I have a huge appetite and eat a corresponding large amount of food.

A tip: Do some experimenting with your mealtimes, with the length of the fasting period, with the number of meals per day. Remember that when humans were still primarily hunters and gatherers, there were no clocks to remind them to eat their meals.

Always on Time?

Our ancestors ate when they had food available to them, but they certainly didn't eat when it was dark; that would have been awkward and dangerous, too. This is true even today: The later you eat your last meal of the day, the worse it is for your overall health. The basic reasons may have changed, but the effect is the same. Thus, if at all possible, try not to eat after 8:00 PM. Rearrange your fasting and eating times as needed, but always try to adhere to an overall fasting period of at least sixteen hours or longer. It's fine if there are days on which you eat only one big meal or fast for up to twenty-two hours. Just don't forget to drink a lot of fluids on these days.

Food Combining

Most foods contain all three major macronutrients—proteins, fats, and carbohydrates—in varying amounts.

Depending on what the foods consist of, the body needs different enzymes to break them down. That is the idea behind "food combining." This system suggests that meals with large amounts of carbohydrates should be eaten in the early afternoon hours and those with more protein in the evening. This allows the pancreas to have a rest, puts less insulin into the bloodstream, and throws the body's switches from growth to "repair and regeneration" (more about this in the section on the three meals on page 91). The recipes in this book were arranged with this principle in mind.

No Snacking!

When I began working as a physician, the word of the day was eating many small meals. And even today, some people still suggest eating five small plant-based meals a day. Diabetics especially are encouraged to eat up to six or even seven meals. But now we know that constant snacking doesn't allow the pancreas to take a break. When we continue to eat, it must keep producing insulin, which effectively opens the floodgates to diabetes.

If the stomach is rarely or never empty, the sirtuins (see page 21) can't start their repair work, causing cell regeneration to grind to a halt. It's all very logical: If you work a lot during the day, you don't continue working into the evening. Instead, you relax and sleep to prepare for the next day. And why should it be different with our organs? They, too, need to take a break sometimes. That is why intermittent fasting is the best, most effective, and most efficient way to strike a balance between action and rest. The bottom line: Don't snack.

The Secret's in the Sum

Our body needs things in moderation. Even an abundance of healthy foods can overtax and thus harm our bodies. Eating an avocado toast or a handful of nuts during the day is good for you; eating a whole loaf of bread or an entire package of nuts is not.

Learn (or relearn) to eat slowly and to chew your food deliberately. If you do, you will soon notice when you have become full. Stomach pains, bloating, and other digestive problems can generally be remedied by regulating the amount we eat on a daily basis. Too much is too much.

Well Chewed = Half Digested

You can assist your digestive system by using your teeth more. Proper chewing stimulates the digestive juices in our mouth that break down our food, especially the carbohydrates.[80] Further, by activating the muscles in our face, chewing increases the blood flow to our entire head, which in turn boosts our brainpower.[81]

Chew as long as you need to, until the food in your mouth has become nearly liquid, and then swallow. The advantage of this method is that you will feel full more quickly—and you will feel less tired and improve your digestion. People generally have poor digestion because they fail to chew their food properly. Why else would we have teeth?

No One Eats the Perfect Diet

No one's diet is 100 percent perfect—there are just too many delightful things out there to eat. And that's OK. Our body is very forgiving, and even the organs that detoxify our bodies need something to do, right? And, of course, sometimes we just need to nourish our soul. So, don't be too hard on yourself: Strict restrictions generally don't work and may even trigger a greater desire for those foods you feel compelled to avoid. Just let them be exceptions, and you'll be fine. Don't feel bad to treat yourself!

What Have You Got to Drink?

Especially in the first fourteen days of intermittent fasting, it's important to drink enough fluids, particularly water. We recommend a daily intake of 85 to 100 ounces (2.5 to 3 liters). The breakdown of body fat, combined with the activation of cell "repair work," means your body is very busy transporting and eliminating toxic metabolic substances. Furthermore, a sufficient amount of water is a prerequisite for nutrients reaching the cells and for getting rid of waste products. That means a lot of water! To best support these processes, we have the following three suggestions:

Fill the Tank in the Morning Hours

Drink a lot in the morning, that is, *before* your first meal of the day—up to 70 ounces (2 liters). This helps your body to eliminate waste products. The best solution is to drink many small portions so that the small intestines can absorb the fluids properly and slowly release them into the body. If you drink too much at once, the water goes directly to the colon, disrupts digestion, and may even cause minerals, like sodium, to be flushed out.[82]

The best thing to drink is spring water, reverse-osmosis filtered water, or pure water with few minerals. If the taste is too boring for you, spice it up by preparing a pitcher in the morning and adding in a few slices of lemon or orange, some fresh mint leaves, lemon balm, or basil. Make it to suit your taste or mood. These additions enhance the taste but will have no influence on your insulin level and thus will not interrupt the fasting period. Alternatively, you can also drink unsweetened tea, best without any milk (plant-based or other) while fasting. During the eating phase, plant-based milk is, of course, allowed. I would particularly recommend the homemade varieties introduced on pages 144 to 146, which contain no additives at all.

Caffeinated coffee and alcohol should be avoided completely, if possible. If you've been drinking coffee on a regular basis, you may suffer from a sort of withdrawal in the first few days without it, accompanied by headaches and nausea, general unwellness, even vomiting. To wean yourself off caffeine a little more gently, try cutting it out ten days before starting your intermittent fasting regimen.

The Secret of Green Tea

Green tea contains many antioxidants, of which the catechins have the greatest beneficial effects. Catechins have both antibacterial and antiviral properties and are responsible for the cancer-inhibiting potential of green tea. One catechin, EGCG (epigallocatechin-3-gallate), is particularly good at preventing and treating arthritis, cancer, diabetes, and obesity.[83]

But not every type of green tea has the same amount of antioxidants. It depends on where it's grown, when it's harvested, how it's produced, and how the tea is brewed. Note the country of origin and whether the tea is organic. The organic label is the only way to ensure that it has been grown without pesticides.

Exercise Moves Nutrients to the Cells

Movement is essential to getting the nutrients to where they can do the most good. Movement is created by our muscles, and our blood flows as the heart pumps it out. The most important transportation system in our body is the bloodstream! Blood carries nutrients to the cells and carries the waste products away. On its own, our heart is unable to get the blood through all of our blood vessels: It needs the help of the venous valves to build up our blood pressure. In the 60,000 miles (100,000 km) of capillaries in our body, where the greatest loss of pressure occurs, tiny layers in the connective tissue assist to ensure proper blood flow. Once the nutrients have gone through the capillary wall and reached the intercellular space, the body can use the flow channels created by the lattice-like structure of the fascia to get nutrients to the cells.

External Movement Creates Internal Movement

In addition to the heart muscle, which is continually in action, the processes described above demand physical movement. Without physical movement, neither the venous valves nor the tiny valves in the capillaries can pump the blood back to the heart. Without movement, the fasciae can develop blockages. And if our connective tissue and bones are not sufficiently stressed through movement, they cannot create the proper electric current necessary to maintain the current in the cell walls. Thus, external physical movement is an absolute prerequisite for all internal movement, namely, to ensure that the nutrients and oxygen reach the cells, and that waste materials are transported to the body's detoxing organs. If you move too little in life, your cells go "hungry," resulting in a buildup of waste in the intercellular space. This, in turn, causes an overall loss of energy and drive as well as a number of lifestyle and chronic diseases (see pages 27 to 39).

Muscles, Our Hormone Factories

In sum, our muscles are responsible for our internal metabolism. But, of course,

they do much, much more. One by-product of muscle movement and contraction is the hormone-like neurotransmitters: the myokines. Currently, we know of some three hundred different myokines, though there are likely many thousands more. These neurotransmitters are decisive in the activation of metabolic processes in the muscles, the liver, and the brain. They ensure that blood vessels are reproduced, that muscles grow, that the structure and function of the brain are secure, that muscles and fat are properly distributed— and they regulate the breakdown of fatty tissues and create an anti-inflammatory environment in the body. Since chronic inflammatory conditions can be the breeding ground for many diseases, the myokines prevent chronic diseases. Thus, the body can only be and remain healthy if it produces enough neurotransmitters to influence its metabolic processes. The motor behind all of these processes is physical movement.

In the next chapter, we explore movement as part of our intermittent fasting method. It's important for everyone to understand that, above and beyond our general everyday movement, special exercises can fire up an explosive effect in your body.

PART TWO

The 14-Day Program

Now that you've learned the benefits of intermittent fasting, you're ready to get started with our fourteen-day food and exercise program.

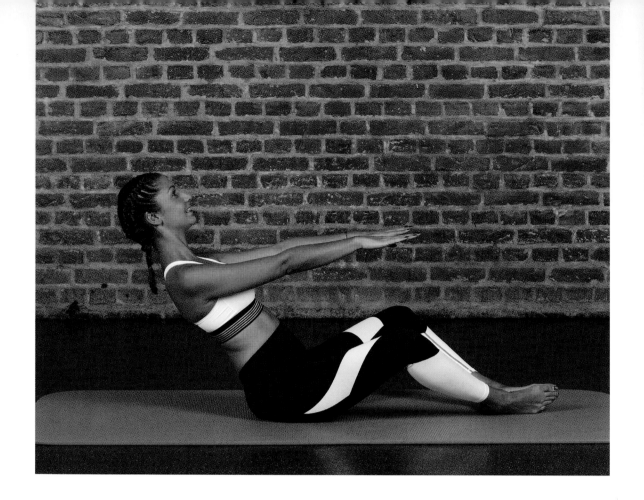

Exercises

Patients who suffer from pain, muscle tension, or signs of physical wear and tear generally get little help from conventional medicine. That changes now! We wanted to discover what exercises would best support efforts at intermittent fasting and return your body to health. To create this exercise regimen, we drew on our thirty-year experience in the development of pain therapy. We discovered a total of twenty-seven problem areas in the muscular-fascial system that are responsible for nearly all tension and pain. Based on these insights, we developed twenty-seven exercises everyone can do to free themselves of pain. Only a pain-free body can best supply the cells with the nutrients they need.

Give your body what it needs to be healthy: endurance, power, muscle control, flexibility, and more. And the easiest way to do that is through exercise! In addition to frequent cardio exercises, we recommend the exercises we developed for just this purpose (see pages 64 to 87).

Cardio Exercises

Any endurance exercise should activate as many muscle groups as possible. Thus, we recommend walking, cross-country skiing, swimming, and rowing, in addition to our exercises, for the best full body workout.

Our Exercise Method

These exercises comprise a very efficient stretching and strength-training program that enables you to systematically eliminate any muscular-fascial issues and movement restrictions, while at the same time ensuring that your muscles release myokines (see page 59), activating your metabolism. Depending on your situation, you can commence endurance training from the beginning or wait until your pain has subsided and your mobility has improved.

BEFORE YOU START

We developed the following exercises to accompany the 14-Day Intermittent Fasting Program. Each day has its own four exercises. If you're able, you should also do cardio endurance training two to three times a week for thirty to forty minutes. Be sure to wear comfortable clothing and sneakers. You may find it helpful to use a yoga mat. Choose a place where you feel relaxed—and try to exercise at the same time every day, if possible. This will help you to establish a routine that makes it easier to continue these exercises for two weeks. Soon, these exercises will become as easy and natural to you as brushing your teeth.

Pelvis Down + Pelvis Up

Letting the pelvis hang down frees you from pain in the lower back, damage caused by overloading the spinal disks, and arthritis in the hip joint. Pulling the pelvis up strengthens the front of the body and stretches the hamstrings, calves, and shoulders.

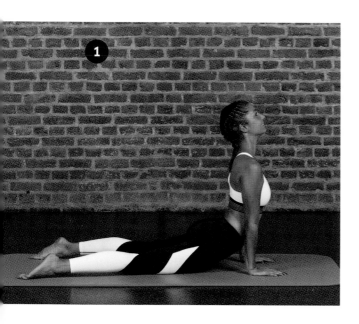

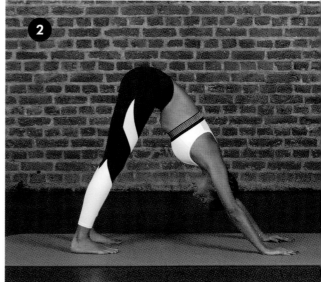

Pelvis Down

▶ Start out on all fours, with your knees directly under your hips. Your arms should be perpendicular to the floor.

▶ **(1)** Press your thighs down against the floor as hard as you can. Hold, then release the tension and let your pelvis sink down just a little bit more. Repeat 40 times, for about 1 minute total.

Pelvis Up

▶ **(2)** Starting from the previous position, press your pelvis up as high as possible, with the legs extended. Try to bring your heels all the way down to the floor. When your pelvis is at its highest, hold for a few counts. Repeat 40 times, for about 1 minute total.

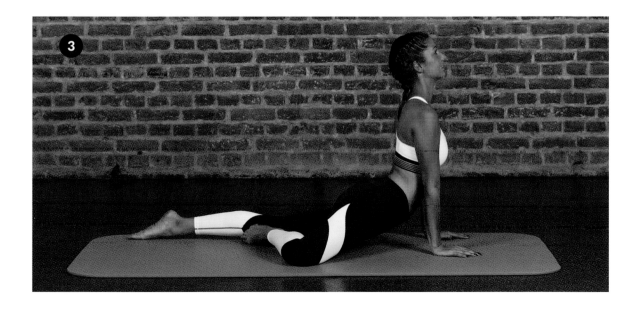

▶ Return your pelvis as quickly as possible to the down position. Do 20 repetitions, moving your pelvis up and down, for about 1 minute.

▶ Sit on your heels and stretch your arms out front and onto the floor. Hold this position for a few deep breaths.

Variation

▶ **(3)** Bend one knee, placing the sole of your foot on the inside of your thigh in the "pelvis down" position. Repeat with the opposite foot.

TRAINING TIPS

• If you find it difficult to hold yourself up on your outstretched arms, do the exercise in an elbow plank position.

• If you discover you don't have the strength to pull your pelvis completely into the upward position, start by going as high as you can.

• If you're unable to complete all of the repetitions, do as many as possible, stopping after the suggested time (1 minute).

• If anything causes pain, stop and take a few days off or reduce the intensity.

Hip Flexor Stretch + Bridge

This exercise strengthens and alleviates pain in the hip joint, buttocks, and lower back and increases flexibility and relieves arthritis in the hip joint.

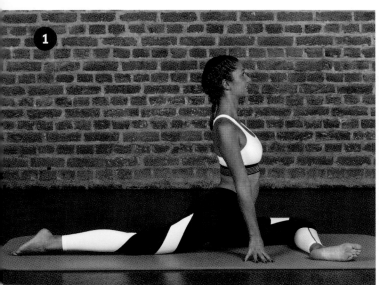
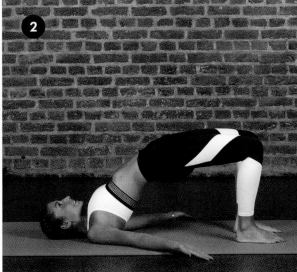

Hip Flexor Stretch

▸ **(1)** Sit on the floor, extend your left leg to the front, and bend your knee as close to a 90-degree angle as possible, but do not tilt your pelvis. Extend your right leg straight behind you as far as possible. The top of your right foot should be pressed against the floor, with the sole facing the ceiling. Your abdomen should be upright and as perpendicular to the floor as possible.

▸ Press your front foot and your back knee against the mat as much as possible. Hold, then release the tension and try to hold your upper body even more perpendicular to the floor.

▸ Repeat 20 times, for about 30 seconds total. Then switch sides and repeat the exercise, for about 30 seconds, with your right leg in front and your left leg behind.

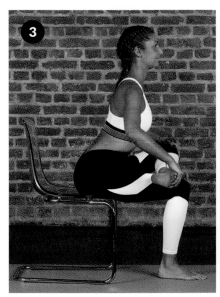

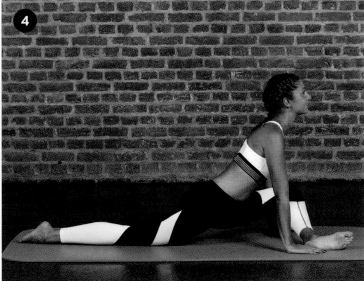

Bridge

▶ **(2)** Begin from a supine position (lying with your back flat on the floor). Bend your knees so that both feet are flat on the floor. Raise your pelvis as high as you can and hold, trying to lift your pelvis just a little bit higher each time. Lower your pelvis to the floor. Repeat 20 times, for about 1 minute total.

Hip Flexor Stretch

▶ Go back to the original hip flexor position. Do this exercise 20 times with your left leg in front, then 20 times with your right leg in front, for about 30 seconds on each side.

Variation 1

▶ **(3)** If doing this exercise on the floor is too difficult for you, sit on a chair, place one leg over your other thigh in a figure-four stretch, and lean forward with your torso as much as possible (your back should be flat) until you feel a strong stretch in your buttocks.

Variation 2

▶ **(4)** If you're already warmed up, you can make the exercise more intense by lifting your buttocks off the floor, balancing with your arms, leaning forward, and raising your pelvis directly up. In this position, the pelvis starts high above the floor. The more you stretch, the more it will sink down.

Spinal Stretch + Sit-Up

This stretching exercise makes the entire back, as well as the neck, buttocks, and legs, more flexible. The sit-ups strengthen the hip flexor and stomach muscles.

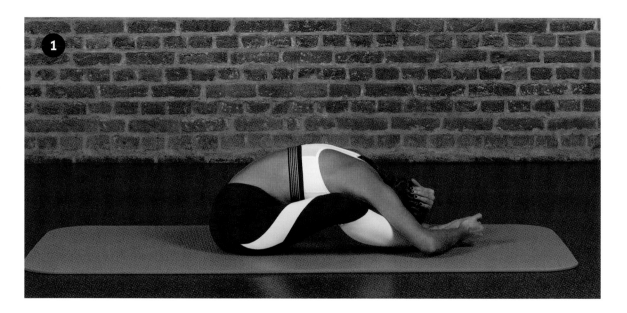

Spinal Stretch

▶ **(1)** Sit on the mat with your legs extended in front of you and bent at about 90 degrees, so that the soles of the feet touch each other. Put your left hand behind your head and grasp the toes of both feet with your right hand. Pull your torso forward as far as possible with your right hand and push your head and upper body down as far as possible with your left hand.

▶ Increase the tension in this position: Flatten your back, push your pelvis down to the floor, and pull your head up. At the point of greatest tension, hold, release the tension, then repeat, increasing the stretch with both hands. Repeat 40 times, for about 1 minute total.

Sit-Up

▶ **(2)** In the supine position (back flat on the floor), bend your legs slightly with the soles of your feet on the ground. Bring your torso up as far as possible and extend your arms out in front of you. As you come up, hold, and then return to the supine position, with your head resting on the mat. Repeat 20 times, for about 1 minute total.

▶ **(3)** Try to extend the stretch by bringing your torso even farther forward with each repetition.

Spinal Stretch

▶ Switch hands and place your right hand behind your head and your left hand on your feet. Pull yourself forward into the spinal stretch.

Variation

▶ If this exercise is too difficult for you and you are unable to grasp your feet easily, use a towel or a yoga strap to help you.

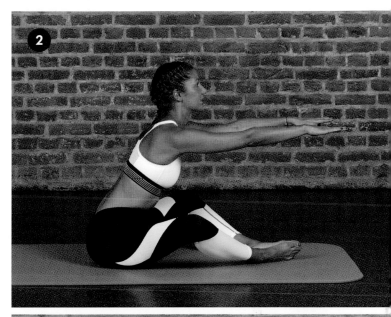

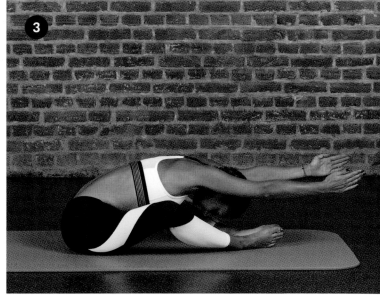

Quad Stretch + Knee Bend

This exercise can prevent—or even get rid of—knee pain, even if you suffer from arthritis or damage to your meniscus or ligaments.

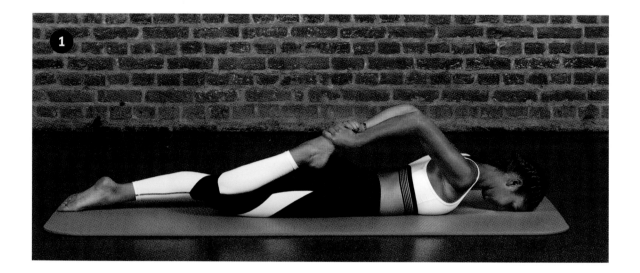

Quad Stretch

▸ **(1)** While lying in the prone position (on your stomach), press your right side to the mat, then place your right hand on the top of the right foot and your left hand on the sole of the right foot. With your hands, pull your foot closer to your buttocks. (If your arms are too short, see the variation that follows.) Continue to press your right side to the mat and stretch. Hold, then release and repeat, pulling the foot to the buttocks. Repeat 20 times for about 30 seconds total.

▸ Switch legs and hands and repeat the exercise, also 20 times.

Variation

▸ If you are unable to grasp your foot with both hands, it may be helpful to "extend" your arms using a towel, a yoga strap, an elastic band, or even a belt. This is important because your entire side should be firmly pressed to the mat *before* you pull your foot to the buttocks.

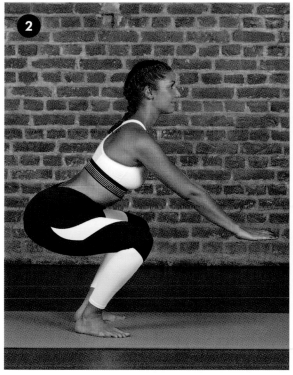

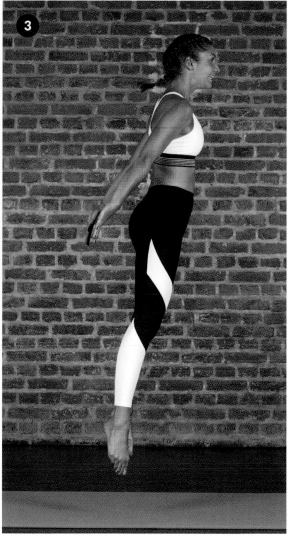

Knee Bend

▶ **(2)** Place your feet squarely on the mat, about shoulder distance apart. Your feet should be slightly turned out. Feel tension through your outer thighs. Bend your knees and lower your pelvis down, as if you were sitting in a chair. Hold your torso as straight as possible by stretching the arms out in front of you. Plant the heels firmly on the mat and hold.

▶ **(3)** Return to the start position and, if possible, jump. If you find jumping difficult, simply straighten your legs. Repeat 20 times for about 1 minute total.

Quad Stretch

▶ Lie once again in the prone position and repeat the exercise first with the right leg and then with the left leg, 30 seconds for each leg.

Hamstring Stretch +
Diagonal Crunch with Leg Raise

Increasing the flexibility of the hamstrings reduces the load on the knees and relieves pain in the knee and the knee hollow (popliteal area). It also helps with damage to the meniscus and lowers the overall risk of cardiovascular diseases.

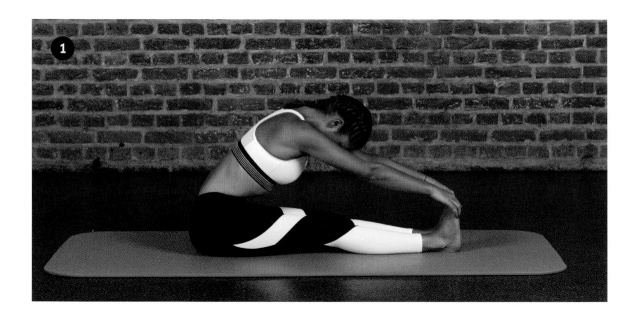

Hamstring Stretch

▶ **(1)** While sitting on the mat, extend your legs to the front, parallel to each other. With a flat back, grab the top of your feet with your hands, a towel, or a yoga strap. Stretch your hamstrings until you can feel it in the back of your knees. Keeping your feet extended, lower your body back to the ground and hold. Relax your whole body, then repeat. Repeat 40 times for about 1 minute total.

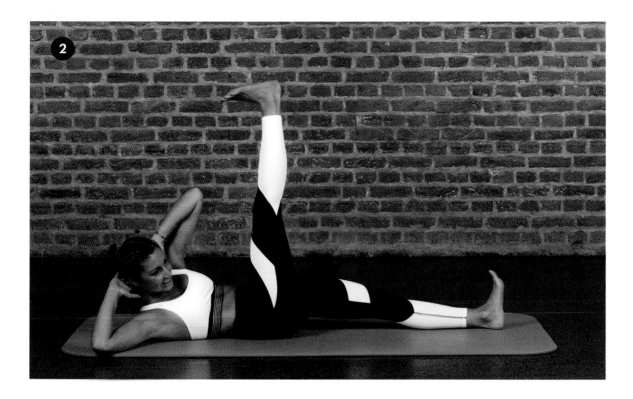

Diagonal Crunch with Leg Raise

▶ **(2)** In the supine position (back flat on the floor), extend your legs. Place your hands behind your head. Pull your extended right leg up into the air as far as possible and touch your left elbow to your right knee. Hold, then lower your leg. Switch legs and repeat. Repeat 20 times for about 1 minute total.

Hamstring Stretch

▶ Sit up once again and repeat the first exercise for about 1 minute.

HELPFUL HINTS

- If need be, use an elastic band, a towel, or a belt to reach your feet and stretch your knees completely while maintaining a straight back (2).

- If the heel of your extended leg lifts slightly from the mat when your knee is being stretched, put a thick book under your heel.

Chest Stretch + Superman

This exercise relieves shoulder pain and helps prevent shoulder impingement syndrome, frozen shoulder (adhesive capsulitis), and arthritis. The rotation reduces tension in the spine. Raising the legs and arms strengthens the back muscles.

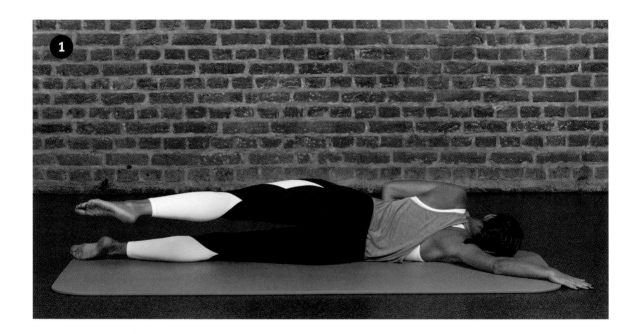

Chest Stretch

▶ **(1)** While lying in the prone position (on your stomach), stretch your right arm out 45 degrees above the shoulder. Press into the ground with your left hand and rotate your whole body onto the right shoulder, so that your right side touches the mat. Press your right arm against the floor and hold. Relax your arm and repeat. Repeat 20 times for about 30 seconds total.

▶ Repeat with your other arm 20 times for about 30 seconds.

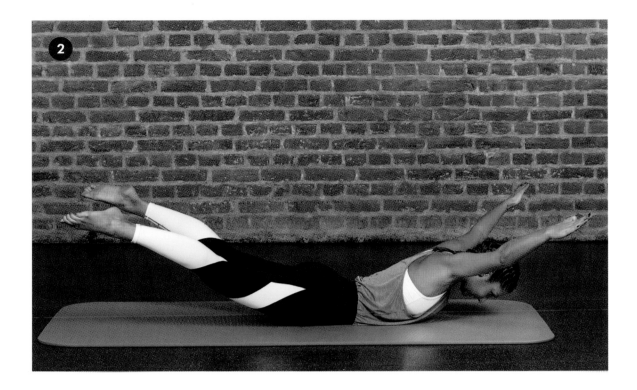

Superman

▶ **(2)** While lying in the prone position, raise both arms and both legs into the air, hold, and then lower down to the mat. Repeat 30 times for about 1 minute total.

Chest Stretch

▶ In the final round, repeat the chest stretch for about 30 seconds on each side.

Variation

▶ If you can't lower your shoulder down to the mat when your arm is at a 45-degree angle, reduce the angle until you can. With each round, try to get closer to the 45-degree angle while leaving your shoulder flat on the ground. If it's difficult for you to raise both legs and both arms at the same time, start with your arms first. As you get stronger, you can add in the legs.

Calf Stretch + Lunge

This exercise relieves tension that can damage the knees. It can also prevent or repair any Baker's cysts and relieve knee pain. Lunges train the knee extensors and buttocks and maintain flexibility in the hip joint.

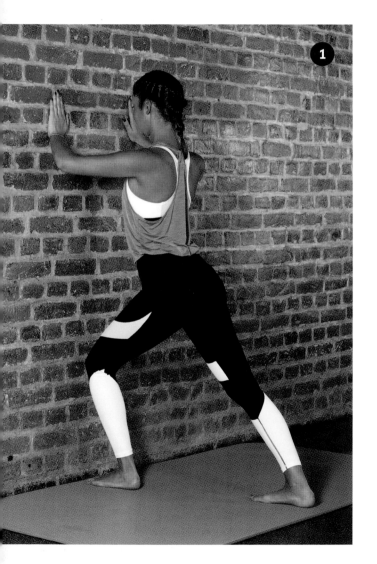

Calf Stretch

▸ **(1)** Stand directly in front of a wall and support yourself by putting your hands against the wall. Move your right foot back about one and a half steps. Your feet should be parallel and pointed toward the wall, and both heels should be pressed against the floor. Bend your left knee until your right leg is fully extended and you feel the stretch in your right calf.

▸ Press the ball of your right foot against the floor and raise your heel, then return to the stretch position and hold. Repeat 20 times for each leg, for about 1 minute total. If no wall is available, this calf stretch can be done without one.

- **For a deeper stretch:** Try tilting your entire torso to the rear, slowly through your hip joint (without creating an arch in your back). This produces an additional strong pull on your right side, stretching your hip extensor as well.

Lunge

- **(2)** Take a big step forward with your right leg and lower your left knee toward the floor.

- **(3)** Straighten your right leg slightly and come up, then go down once again. If that's too difficult for you, extend your right leg more or even completely. Repeat 10 times per leg, for about 1 minute total.

- If you don't have enough strength to carry through with the lunge, don't go all the way down to the floor, but do try to get lower with each repetition. As your legs become stronger, extend the front leg less and less, leaving it permanently bent at a 90-degree angle.

Calf Stretch

- Repeat the calf stretch for 30 seconds for each leg.

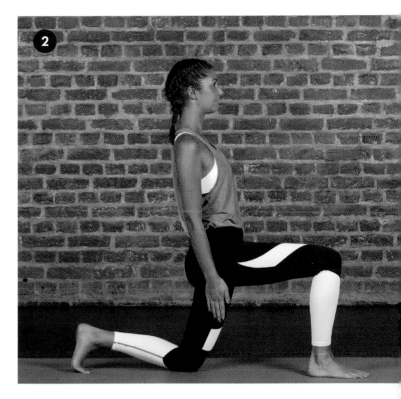

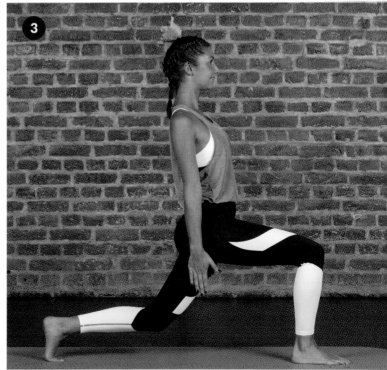

Tricep Stretch + Push-Up

This is the ideal exercise for people with shoulder pain. It also helps if you have calcification in the shoulder, a frozen shoulder, or shoulder impingement syndrome, and it can prevent shoulder joint arthritis. It strengthens and stabilizes the whole shoulder area.

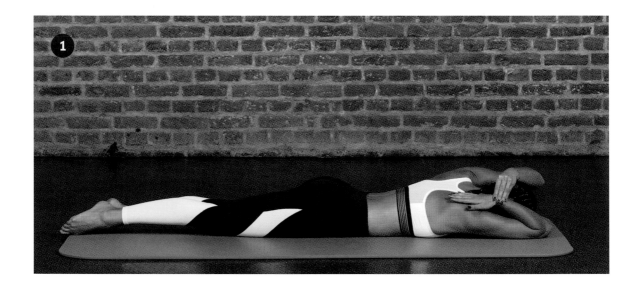

Tricep Stretch

▶ **(1)** While lying in the prone position (on your stomach), extend your right arm to the front, then bend your elbow so that your right hand comes to lie on your right shoulder. Place the fingers of your left hand on your right wrist. Press your right armpit and your right elbow to the mat, press your right hand upward against your left hand, and hold.

▶ Release, then repeat 20 times for about 1 minute total. Repeat 20 times on the other side for about 1 minute.

▶ If lying in the prone position is unpleasant for you, try the tricep exercise while standing against a wall.

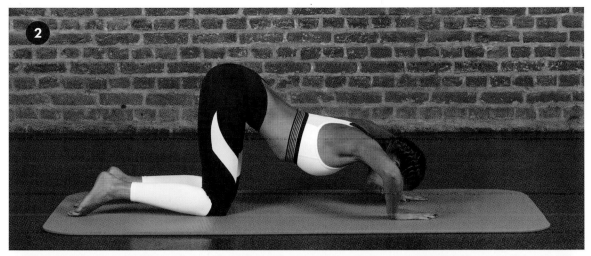

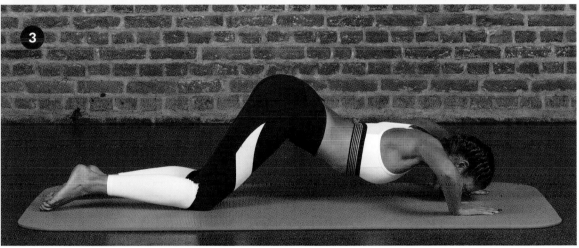

Push-Up

▶ **(2)** Start out on all fours, with your knees directly under your hips. Your arms should be perpendicular to the floor. Bend your arms and lower your upper body to the floor, touching your nose to the mat. Lower your upper body slowly, then press your upper body up again until your arms are completely extended. Repeat 30 times for about 30 seconds total. If your knees hurt, try putting a blanket or a towel under them.

▶ **(3)** For a more challenging push-up, move your hands farther forward. You can also start in a plank position for the most challenging variation.

Tricep Stretch

▶ Return to the prone position and repeat this exercise.

Neck Stretch + Tabletop

This exercise relieves excess tension in the cervical spine, which is responsible for overextension. It also eliminates headache and neckache and prevents spinal disk damage. The backwards push-up opens the shoulders and strengthens the back and buttocks.

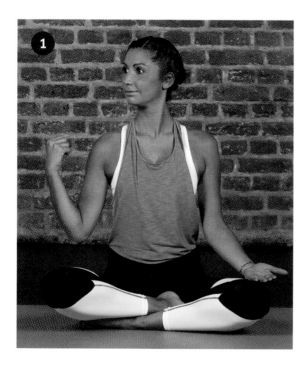

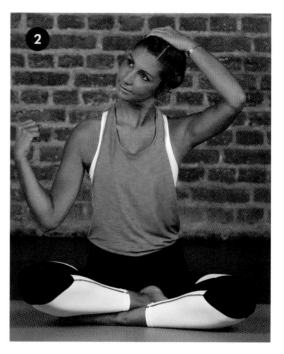

Neck Stretch

▶ **(1)** Sit on the floor or in a chair in a comfortable position. Straighten both your lumbar spine and your thoracic spine by extending your breastbone forward. Now turn your head 45 degrees to the right. Bend your right elbow and pull your right shoulder down as far as possible.

▶ **(2)** Raise your left hand above your head and pull your head very carefully to the side. You can increase the tension by pressing your head against your left hand.

▶ Repeat the sequence 20 times for about 30 seconds total, then change sides and repeat 20 times for an additional 30 seconds.

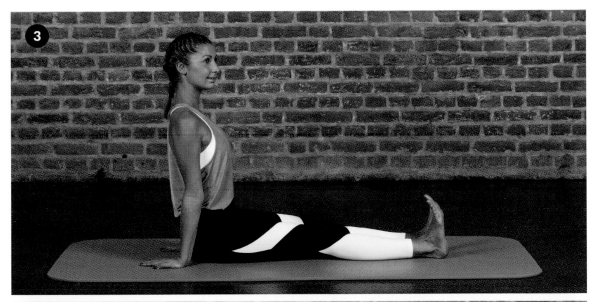

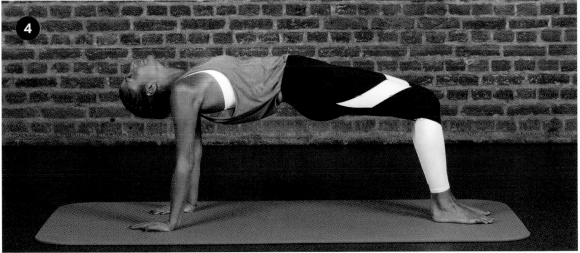

Tabletop

▶ **(3)** Sit on the floor with your legs stretched out in front of you, your arms perpendicular to the floor, and your hands at your side with your palms on the floor, fingers facing back.

▶ **(4)** Raise your pelvis up and to the front, then extend your head to the rear. Straighten your cervical spine. Repeat 20 times for about 1 minute.

Neck Stretch

▶ Repeat the neck stretch for 30 seconds on each side.

Full Body Stretch + Side Plank

This exercise stretches the sides of the body. This gets rid of pain in the back (lumbosciatica) and hip joints as well as any pain in the outsides of the legs and knees. The side plank strengthens and stretches the side body.

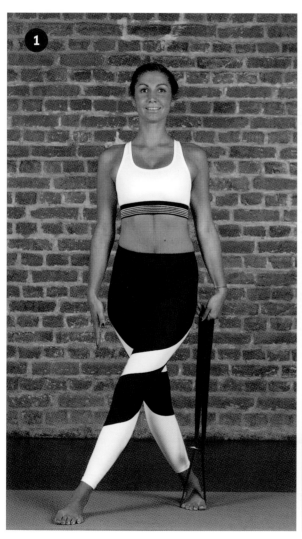

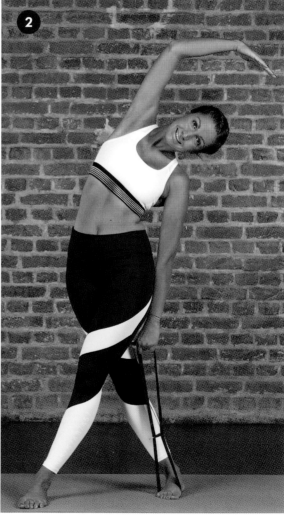

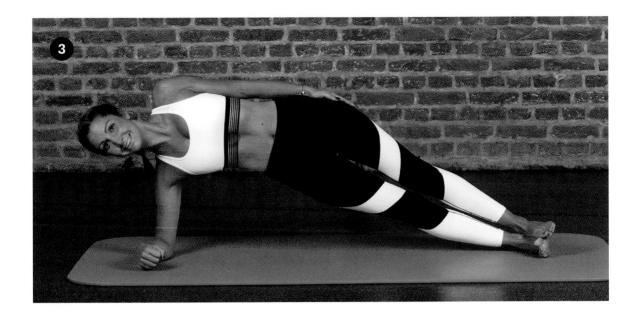

Full Body Stretch

▶ **(1)** While standing, hold an elastic band in your right hand and insert your right foot into it. Pass the elastic band through your legs over to your left hand and move your right foot behind your left leg as far as possible (a "curtsy").

▶ **(2)** Increase the stretch by pulling the band farther to the left and moving your right arm up and over your head.

▶ Repeat 20 times, pulling against the band, feeling the resistance, and releasing. This should take about 30 seconds total. Repeat 20 times on the other side.

▶ If it's difficult for you to hold your balance, hold on to something with one hand: a wall, a table, or the back of a chair.

Side Plank

▶ **(3)** Lie on your right side, then place your right elbow on the floor, directly under your right shoulder. Place your left foot on top of your right foot and lift your pelvis up as far as possible. Hold, then release the tension and return your pelvis to the mat (3). Repeat 20 times for about 30 seconds.

▶ If you can't hold the side plank, brace yourself with one hand or leave your upper leg on the floor until you have gained enough strength. To increase the difficulty, place your right hand flat on the floor, directly under your right shoulder, and lift, straightening your right arm.

Full Body Stretch

▶ Repeat the exercise again on both sides.

Shoulder-Chest Stretch + Hip Dips

This exercise eliminates any remaining tension in the shoulders and side body. It gets rid of shoulder pain and increases shoulder flexibility. The plank stabilizes the shoulders and strengthens the abdominal muscles.

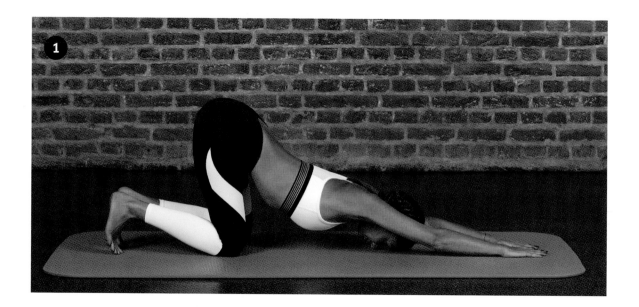

Shoulder-Chest Stretch

▶ **(1)** On all fours, walk your hands to the front of the mat until your elbows are locked and your thighs are perpendicular to the floor. Lower your breastbone toward the floor so that your thumbs meet in the middle. Move your breastbone back toward your knees until you can feel the stretch in your shoulders.

▶ Increase the tension by pushing your hands as hard as possible against the floor. Release the tension and then repeat.

▶ Do a total of 40 repetitions for about 1 minute total.

Hip Dips

▶ **(2)** Start in a forearm plank position. Turn your pelvis to the right and

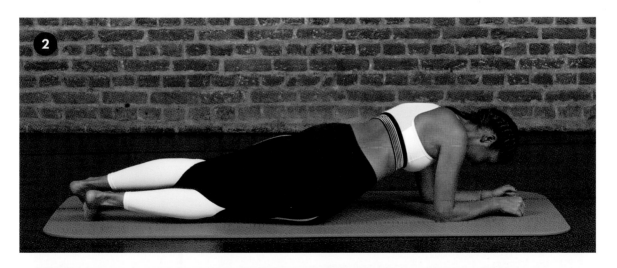

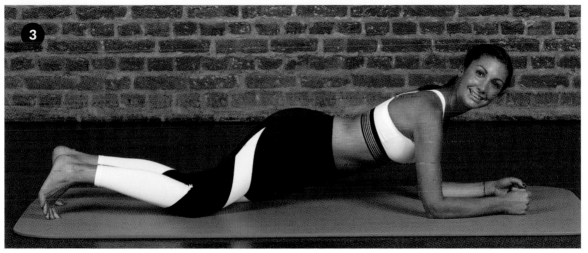

lower it to the mat, then raise it, turn it to the left, and lower it to the mat. Turn to the right and hold, then turn to the left and hold. Repeat 40 times for about 1 minute.

▶ **(3)** If you find it difficult to keep your body elevated in plank position, support yourself on your knees until you build up strength. If you begin on the tips of your feet and then have to

stop because your body isn't stable enough, rest on your knees and keep going.

Shoulder-Chest Stretch

▶ Go once again to the all-fours position and repeat the stretch. Do 40 repetitions for about 1 minute.

Rotation Stretches

This exercise relieves pain in the feet, knees, hip joints, spine, neck, and head.

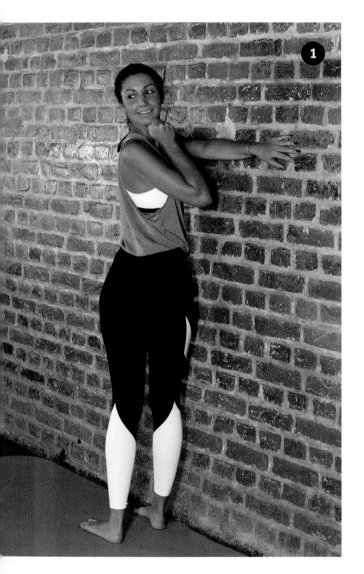

Rotation 1

▶ **(1)** Stand sideways with your right shoulder against a wall; your weight should be equally distributed between both feet. Put your left palm on the wall and place your right index finger on the left side of your lower jaw.

▶ Using both hands, rotate your torso and your head to the right as far as you can. To increase the tension, try to turn your torso and head even farther to the right and hold. Relax and stretch. Repeat this exercise 20 times for about 30 seconds total. Switch sides and repeat 20 times for the left side, for about 30 seconds.

Rotation 2

▶ **(2)** Stand with your feet about shoulder-width apart. Extend your right arm out to the side and place your left hand on your chest. Rotate your torso as far as possible to the right; your head should turn, too. Hold, then release.

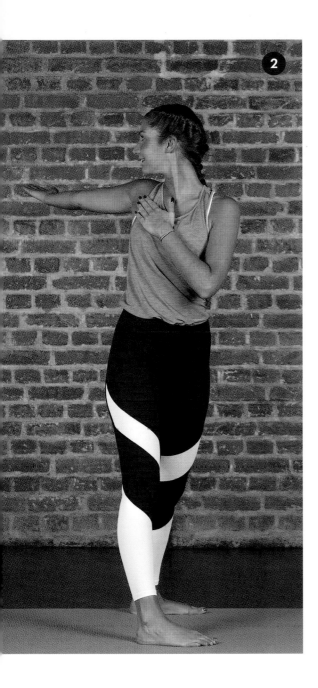

▸ Change the direction and turn to the left. Do a total of 40 repetitions, alternating between left and right rotations, for about 1 minute.

Rotation 1

▸ Resume the position against the wall and repeat Rotation 1. Do a total of 40 repetitions for about 1 minute.

FULL BODY ROTATION

Your hips should rotate completely as far as your feet and knee joints allow. This movement can be supported by allowing your gaze to follow your arms. Pay close attention to your breathing: Inhaling and exhaling should run parallel to—not contrary to—the rotation movements and always in the same rhythm.

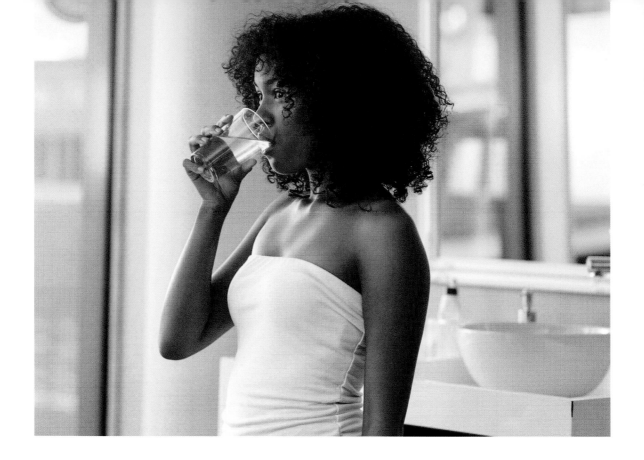

How to Start
Intermittent Fasting

Changing your eating habits may seem daunting, but it's 100 percent worth it. And how you begin is, of course, up to you. Perhaps you want to try it out for a couple of days at first, or only from Monday to Friday, or only on the weekends. Or you can commit to eating this way every day from the start. Our 14-Day Program is the perfect way to start. If you choose to begin your intermittent fasting with this program, I recommend that you stick closely to it for the first fourteen days. After that, you can introduce a little more variation in your daily routines. And over time, you will develop an instinct for what is good for you—and what is not.

Before You Start

How quickly your body gets used to the new eating schedule depends greatly on your lifestyle. There's no hard-and-fast rule that says how quickly someone will become hungry. Many factors play a role in this: how much you exercise, your previous diet, and your mental state. Even the time of the year or the weather can influence things.

But the wonderful thing is: There's no pressure. Don't be afraid to just try it out. With a few short tips and tricks for getting started, everyone can be on their way to intermittent fasting. There's no major prep work involved. The best thing is to just get started—today!

How It Works

The following recommendations are based on the most frequently asked questions my patients pose when beginning intermittent fasting. Generally speaking, they are mostly little things, but they can be decisive when launching into your own fasting program.

Escaping Hunger

Eat your last meal of the day early in the evening and then go to bed early! Those two things will help you most when you start your fasting program. After three days, at the latest, you will no longer be hungry in the morning.

After the first five days, you will notice that your stomach has become a little flatter. You will also feel more awake and fit, your skin and eyes clearer. The feeling of hunger will disappear a little more every day. Above all, you'll experience how easy it is to extend the time between meals.

Meal Breaks

Plan your meal breaks at the beginning carefully, always listening to your body. Don't start right off with a fasting period of twenty hours; work slowly and deliberately on extending the time. Start with a twelve-hour fast, then increase it by one hour each day. The longer you can extend the fasting time, the better.

Drink Plenty of Fluids

Drink plenty and regularly, especially during the fasting period. A warm cup of tea is a good way to satisfy hunger between meals.

Don't Count Calories

There's no need to count calories. You can eat as much and as many vegetable dishes as you want. The recipes in this book are laid out for two people. If you're very physically active, you may want to interpret "serves 2" as "serves 1." The important thing is: With intermittent fasting you do not need to starve yourself. Rather, the key lies in eating until you are full.

Eating Out

Do you want to eat out or enjoy a meal with friends? No problem! Eating should be fun, and the social aspect of eating a meal, even while adhering to intermittent fasting, is really important. If your goal is to better or to maintain your health, strive to avoid fast food and other obviously unhealthy choices.

Instead, be "picky"—choose soups, vegetables, and salads that you like and that are healthy; choose restaurants that offer healthy, vegetable-forward menus; set up your meals with others during your personal eating intervals to avoid breaking your fasting rhythm.

Start on the Weekend

Take your time. Start on a weekend and prep meals for the coming week, if possible. This way, you'll always have food at the ready for when you need it.

Find a Partner

Try to find a partner who is also interested in starting intermittent fasting. Personal experience shows that sharing things with someone else can be extremely motivating. If you are still skeptical, try seeing intermittent fasting as a challenge for a set period. That might make it easier.

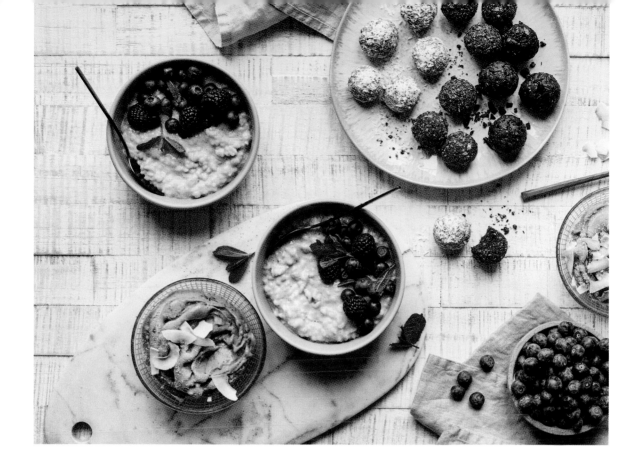

The Three Meals

The First Meal

The first meal after the fasting period should be as healthy as possible. While fasting, your body absorbs nutrients, vitamins, minerals, and phytochemicals efficiently. The perfect sources of energy for your "break-fast" are soft foods of all types, like smoothies made of fresh fruit and leafy green vegetables, and whole-grain foods. Their texture enables digestion to proceed slowly and gently. The first meal of the day is important because you do not want to overtax your stomach and intestine from the start.

The recipes present numerous alternatives that can help to detox your body, while also increasing the positive effects of intermittent fasting. These three simple rules are crucial:

1) *Eat lots of fiber.* Fruits and whole-grain foods not only make you feel full, but they also keep you fit.

2) *Don't start off with sugary foods.* Processed granolas and cereals generally have a lot of added sugar. If you have a sweet tooth, try to prepare your own breakfast and integrate the natural sugars via fruits.

3) *The key is in the quantity.* Don't overtax your digestive system right off the bat, as that may make you tired and sluggish.

When Should You Eat?

For most people who work outside the home, it is easiest to make the eating interval coincide with your work schedule. Thus, the first meal of the day is a true "break-fast," for example, around 9:00 AM. Around noon is the second meal of the day, and the third meal should take place no later than 5:00 PM, if you are to maintain the intermittent fasting rhythm.

But you can be flexible with your fasting times. The first meal of the day need not necessarily be a classical breakfast. For example, if you prefer to start eating at around noon, then you can combine two meals into one (a "brunch" of sorts). That means starting off with, say, a smoothie, so as not to overtax the digestive system, and then adding a second meal thirty to sixty minutes later. The third and last meal is then eaten in the early evening. Another alternative for eating a "late" breakfast: Begin to eat around 1:00 PM with a recipe from the Breakfast chapter (see page 138). The second meal follows at 4:00 PM, and the third between 7:00 PM and 8:00 PM. You should finish eating by 9:00 PM.

The Second Meal

You will likely start to get hungry again about three to four hours after the first meal of the day. But don't adhere to the clock! Wait for your body to signal its needs and try to differentiate between appetite and hunger. A tip: If you are uncertain, drink a large glass of water and then "listen to your body." With a little practice, you will be able to recognize what your body is trying to tell you. Hunger is the signal that your body needs energy. Take the time to nourish it.

Fit Through the Day

The second meal of the day has one main goal: to keep your energy level up and your body supplied with carbohydrates and fiber. This prevents your blood sugar level from rising, satiates hunger, and keeps your energy at a constant level. Regardless of whether you have a job that is physically demanding or sit all day at a desk: You need energy for your brain to work properly.

The Third Meal

The third and final meal of the day should contain lots of protein. First, the body needs less energy during nighttime rest than during the day, when we're more active. Second, at night, the body is occupied with a number of regeneration processes that require amino acids.

Proteins also get the metabolism up and running. They act more slowly and need less insulin than other nutrients. It's not surprising that protein-rich meals are more valuable in the evening hours. You can get an extra protein kick by scattering a few hemp seeds, soy flakes, or a little tofu over any meal.

Eat Earlier

For your body to have enough time to digest your last meal before bedtime, you should try to eat by 6:00 PM, at the very latest by 8:00 PM. The ideal dinner meal is one with few calories, few carbohydrates, and lots of protein. Taking a walk after the evening meal also helps to ensure a pleasant night's sleep. It allows the body to relax, kicks off the burning of fat, and initiates the cleanup and repair work. A positive side effect: If your stomach is empty when you go to bed and your nighttime temperature is lowered, the antiaging enzymes become active (see page 20).

Eating Raw Food in the Evening

Do you sometimes have the feeling that raw foods don't agree with you in the evening? You're not alone, as this happens to many people. However, the cause lies less in the fresh foods themselves than in the carbohydrates and sugars that are consumed at the same time or later. This combination in the evening can trigger strong fermentation processes in the intestine that can be unpleasant.

Combine as few ingredients as possible and, above all, do not consume sugar or sugary foods in the evening, to allow your intestine to concentrate on digesting the raw foods. Here, too, it's important to thoroughly chew your food before swallowing. Try to consume any raw foods earlier in the day, long before you go to bed—ideally at least four hours before.

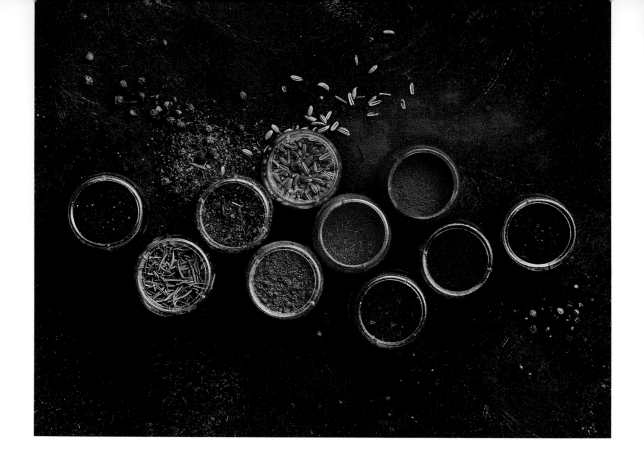

Our Favorite Foods for Intermittent Fasting

For this book, we put together recipes that supply your body with all the nutrients it needs. In the end, that's the most important thing to prevent you from getting hungry during fasting times. It's also the way we cook ourselves. The foods we suggest here are also found on our own refrigerator and pantry shelves.

Our favorite nuts and seeds

Almonds: rich in vitamins B and E; can be used to produce almond milk or almond butter, or eaten as a snack.

Brazil nuts: Three Brazil nuts a day provide all the selenium you need (this essential trace element is often neglected).

Cashews: a super ingredient in the vegan diet; perfect for snacks, as a topping, for sauces, or in self-made cashew milk; contains a healthy portion of zinc and magnesium.

Walnuts: contain many omega-3 fatty acids and are thus a superfood for the brain; can be eaten as a snack or in salads.

Chia seeds: The jelly-like texture of soaked chia seeds is great for your digestion, and the seeds are rich in important omega-3 fatty acids to boot.

Flaxseeds: an excellent source of omega-3 fatty acids; best eaten when freshly milled.

Hemp seeds: a fantastic source of protein, rich in omega-3 fatty acids; best crushed or milled as part of granola or as a topping for bowls and salads.

Sesame seeds: rich in calcium, with a nutty flavor; available either in white or black—the darker the seeds, the greater the amount of nutrients.

Our favorite fats, oils, and vinegars

Canola oil: an excellent, versatile oil, especially because of its ratio of omega-6 to omega-3 fatty acids.

Coconut oil: good for sautéing and for preparing curries and healthy sweets.

Flaxseed oil: our favorite for salad dressings.

Olive oil: the most versatile oil, for dressings, hummus, dips, sauces; can even be used to fry foods, if the temperature is not too high.

Sesame oil: ideal for Asian dishes and dressings.

Apple cider vinegar: used in dressings; is antibacterial and anti-inflammatory.

White balsamic vinegar: brings freshness to any salad dressing.

White wine vinegar: used in sauces and dressings; always fits.

Our favorite (pseudo) grains

Brown rice: the husk is where the nutrients reside, as well as B vitamins, iron, magnesium, and antioxidants.

Buckwheat: an excellent source of protein, great in hearty bowls and in sweet porridges.

Oats: basic component of oatmeal and overnight oats; contains healthy fiber for digestion.

Quinoa: a protein-rich superfood for both savory and sweet dishes.

Wild rice: has many vitamins, minerals, and trace elements.

Our favorite herbs and spices

Cardamom: considered the "queen" of Ayurvedic cuisine; among other things, promotes digestion.

Cayenne pepper: contains capsaicin, a well-known fat-burner; also thins the blood and protects the stomach lining.

Cinnamon: warms the body and regulates blood sugar.

Coriander: supports "cleanup" activities in the body and provides many valuable phytochemicals.

Cumin: a well-known healing herb that helps with digestive problems, particularly distension and bloating.

Curry powder: anti-inflammatory.

Fennel seeds: antibacterial and relaxing.

Sea salt: if natural and untreated, is rich in minerals and trace elements.

Turmeric: anti-inflammatory and analgesic.

Our favorite legumes

Beluga lentils: crispy and crunchy; ideal for salads and as a side dish.

Chickpeas: an excellent source of protein; packed full of magnesium, iron, and copper.

Lentils (yellow, red, brown): rich in protein and fiber; the main ingredient in Indian dals, many salads, and stews.

Our favorite sugar alternatives

Coconut sugar: allows the blood sugar to rise slowly compared to household sugar; has a fine taste.

Dates: our favorite sweet fruit—the juicy Medjool dates are the best.

Maple syrup: excellent for dressings and sweet dishes.

Our favorite fresh ingredients

- Apples
- Avocados
- Bananas
- Carrots
- Fennel
- Garlic
- Ginger
- Herbs
- Lemons
- Lettuce
- Onions
- Oranges
- Potatoes
- Radicchio
- Scallions
- Spinach
- Turmeric
- Zucchini

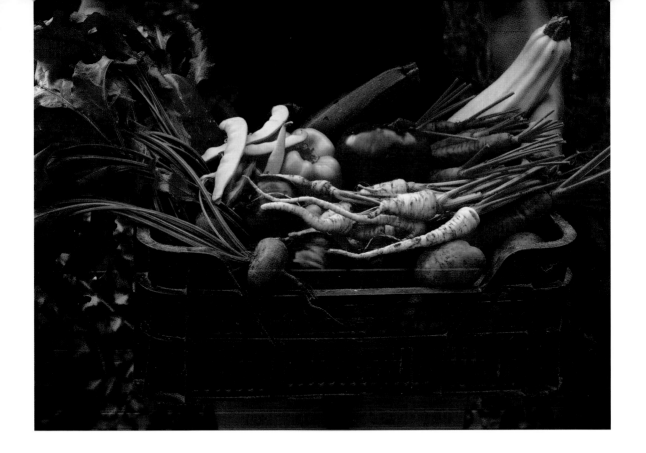

The 14-Day Shopping List

To enable you to better plan your new diet, here is a shopping list for the first two weeks of fasting.

Staples for the 14-Day Program

Pantry

- Agave syrup
- Almond milk (see page 145 to make your own)
- Almonds, whole and sliced
- Amaranth, puffed
- Apple juice
- Cashews
- Chia seeds

- Chickpeas
- Coconut, shredded
- Coconut milk
- Coconut water
- Cornichons
- Cranberries, dried
- Cranberry juice
- Flaxseeds
- Glass noodles (bean thread vermicelli)
- Goji berries
- Hazelnuts
- Lentils, beluga and brown
- Maple syrup
- Millet
- Oats, rolled
- Pine nuts
- Pumpkin seeds
- Quinoa, white and multicolored
- Rice, brown and black
- Rice milk
- Rice noodles, wide
- Sauerkraut

- Sesame seeds, white and black
- Soy milk
- Tofu (silken, firm, and smoked)
- Vegetable broth (see page 174 to make your own)
- Walnuts
- Wild rice

Spices

- Black pepper
- Cacao nibs
- Capers
- Cayenne pepper
- Cinnamon
- Cumin, ground
- Curry powder
- Fennel seeds
- Garam masala
- Ginger, ground
- Marjoram
- Mustard, regular and Dijon

- Nutmeg
- Oregano
- Raw cacao powder
- Sea salt
- Soy sauce
- Sriracha
- Thyme
- Turmeric
- Vanilla beans (or organic vanilla extract)

Vinegars and Oils

- Apple cider vinegar
- Balsamic vinegar
- Canola oil
- Coconut oil
- Hazelnut oil
- Olive oil, regular and extra virgin
- Rice vinegar
- White balsamic vinegar
- White vinegar

Produce for the 14-Day Program

The healthiest and most sustainable diet contains fresh, plant-based, organically farmed foods, locally grown, if possible. That means we should always try to buy fresh foods! To make planning your meals easier, we have prepared a produce shopping list for the first two weeks of fasting.

Week 1

FRUITS

6 lemons

3 apples

3 bananas

3 mangos

3 oranges

2 pears

2 limes

1 grapefruit

10 ounces (280 g) blueberries (fresh and/or frozen)

10 ounces (280 g) strawberries (fresh and/or frozen)

9 ounces (255 g) raspberries (fresh and/or frozen)

7 ounces (200 g) grapes

5½ ounces (150 g) honeydew melon

VEGETABLES

2 pounds (1 kg) waxy potatoes

14 ounces (400 g) baby spinach

14 ounces (400 g) cherry tomatoes (24 total)

10½ ounces (300 g) mixed tomatoes

8 carrots

6 red onions

5 button mushrooms

4 large beefsteak tomatoes

4 mini bell peppers

3 garlic cloves

3 avocados

2 cucumbers

2 eggplants

2 fennel bulbs

2 scallions

2 bunches parsley

2 bunches radishes

2 handfuls cilantro

1 bunch dill

1 bunch mint

1 bunch watercress

2 handfuls micro watercress

1 handful basil

1 handful broccoli florets

1 handful shredded red cabbage

1 kohlrabi

1 bell pepper

1 ginger root (for both weeks)

1 head radicchio

1 large sweet potato

1 small tomato

3½ ounces (100 g) edamame pods

3½ ounces (100 g) sun-dried tomatoes

Week 2

FRUITS

18 ounces (500 g) mixed berries

7 lemons

4 bananas

4 limes

4 oranges

4 pears

2 apples

2 figs

2 mangos

1 kiwi

¼ pineapple

3 ounces (85 g)
    pomegranate seeds

VEGETABLES

2½ pounds (1.1 kg) Yukon
    Gold potatoes

1½ pounds (680 g) carrots

1 pound 5 ounces (600 g)
    baby spinach

6 beets

6 cherry tomatoes

5 red onions

5 beefsteak tomatoes

4 mini bell peppers

3 avocados

2 bell peppers

2 heads broccoli
    (1 pound/500 g each)

2 cucumbers

2 heads radicchio

2 scallions

2 bunches cilantro

2 bunches mint

2 handfuls watercress

1 bunch basil

2 bunches parsley

1 banana pepper

1 large carrot

2 celery roots

1 head garlic

1 small red kuri squash or
    ½ small butternut squash

2 leeks

1 yellow onion

1 zucchini

½ parsley root or celery
    root

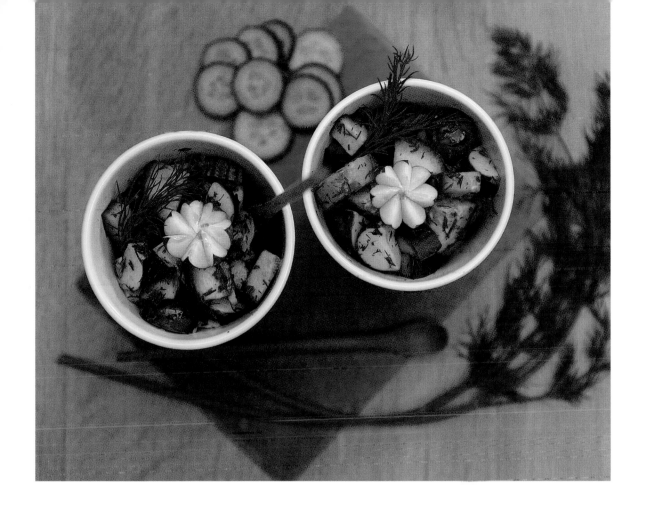

14 Days of Vegan Recipes

Day 4
Tropical Smoothie Bowl
Sweet Potato Coconut Curry
Parsley Salad with Amaranth

Day 5
Quinoa-Berry Porridge
Fried Eggplant with Capers
Tomato and Melon Salad

Day 6
Apple-Cinnamon Overnight Oats
Potato Salad
Rainbow Mason Jar Salad

Day 7
Rainbow Fruit Salad
Wild Rice and Fennel Stir-Fry
Fresh Cucumber and Radish Salad

Day 8
Avocado-Berry Bowl
Glass Noodle Salad
Broccoli and Zucchini Stir-Fry

Day 9
Red Power Smoothie
Chickpea and Spinach Curry
Beet and Radicchio Carpaccio

Day 10
Coconut Millet Porridge
Zucchini Noodles with Tofu and Avocado
Spanish Tomato Salad

Day 11
Berry Chia Bowl
Citrusy Squash Salad
Smoked Tofu and Lentil Stew

Day 12
Energy Smoothie
Black Rice with Mint and Citrus
Colorful Minestrone

Day 13
Strawberry Overnight Oats
Potato Soup
Sauerkraut and Pear Salad with
    Smoked Tofu

Day 14
Banana-Chocolate Chia Pudding
Avocado and Mango Salad
Carrot-Ginger Soup

TIPS FOR GETTING STARTED

Eat What You Want

You can do some reshuffling of the recipes if you want. For example, if on Day 7 you're craving the Buddha Bowl again (see page 104), make it instead of the Fresh Cucumber and Radish Salad (see page 117).

Get Moving

Intermittent fasting is not meant to keep you from moving. Many people think that they will become weaker if they fast, and that they must therefore "take it easy." Actually, the opposite is true! Nutrients get to their destinations more quickly, and waste products exit the body more rapidly, as long as you see to it that your metabolism and blood circulation are working at a brisk pace. That is why we recommend reserving a fixed part of (almost) every day during the 14-Day Program for doing our physical exercises. Plan to do this for at least fifteen minutes every day. If you also do cardio training two or three times a week, your two-week intermittent fasting trial will be a complete success.

Now you're ready to start your new life!

Today is the first day of your completely new life! It starts with a tasty smoothie to melt those extra pounds away. Lunch is a simple Buddha bowl, and you'll end your day with some refreshing raw veggies. On Day 1, we recommend exercises that focus on the abs, upper arms, chest, buttocks, and neck.

Green Smoothie

SERVES 2
PREP TIME: 10 minutes
PER SERVING: 197 calories, 5 g protein, 7 g fat, 22 g carbohydrates

1 apple
1 grapefruit
½ avocado
½ lemon
7 ounces (200 g) baby spinach

1. Core the apple, then cut into quarters. Peel the grapefruit, avocado, and lemon, and cut into small pieces.

2. Place all of the ingredients in a blender with 1⅔ cups (400 ml) water and blend at high speed.

3. Pour into two glasses and enjoy.

Buddha Bowl

SERVES 1
PREP TIME: 20 minutes
PER SERVING: 665 calories, 22 g protein, 23 g fat, 80 g carbohydrates

3 medium waxy potatoes
Sea salt
1 carrot
½ avocado
1 handful watercress
1 handful broccoli florets
1 handful shredded red cabbage
1 tablespoon sliced almonds

DRESSING
3½ ounces (100 g) silken tofu
Juice of 1 lemon
2 tablespoons agave syrup
1 tablespoon mustard
1 teaspoon black sesame seeds
Fresh ground black pepper

1. Peel and cut the potatoes in quarters. Transfer to a medium pot, cover with salted water, and bring to a boil. Cover and let simmer for 5 to 8 minutes, until fork tender. Drain and set aside.

2. While the potatoes cook, cut the carrot into sticks and peel and slice the avocado.

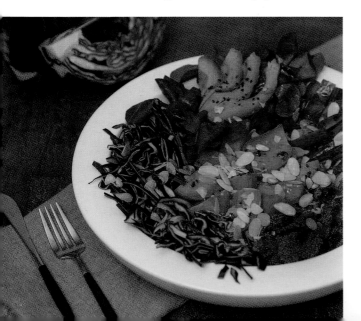

3. Arrange the vegetables in a bowl: Place the potatoes in the middle and scatter the watercress, carrot, broccoli, and cabbage around them. Place the avocado slices on top of the watercress.

4. To make the dressing, mix the tofu, lemon juice, agave syrup, mustard, and sesame seeds in a small bowl. Season with salt and pepper.

5. Pour the dressing over the vegetables, sprinkle the almonds on top, and serve.

Crudité Plate with Guacamole

SERVES 2
PREP TIME: 15 minutes
PER SERVING: 249 calories, 5 g protein, 13 g fat, 21 g carbohydrates

3 carrots
1 kohlrabi
1 bunch radishes
1 bell pepper

GUACAMOLE
1 avocado
Juice of 1 lemon
1 medium tomato
Sea salt
Fresh ground black pepper

1. Peel and julienne the carrots and kohlrabi. Cut the greens off the radishes and cut the radishes in half. Halve the pepper, remove the seeds, and cut into strips. Arrange on a serving plate.

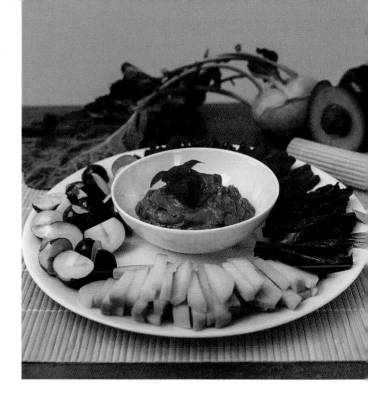

2. To make the guacamole, pit and peel the avocado and place in a food processor or blender with the lemon juice. Pulse until smooth. Finely dice the tomato and stir into the guacamole. Season with salt and pepper.

3. Transfer the guacamole to a small bowl and serve with the vegetables.

TODAY'S EXERCISES

EXERCISE 1:
Pelvis Down + Pelvis Up (page 64)

EXERCISE 2:
Hip Flexor Stretch + Bridge (page 66)

EXERCISE 8:
Tricep Stretch + Push-Up (page 78)

EXERCISE 9:
Neck Stretch + Tabletop (page 80)

Tonight you'll go to sleep feeling great, since, slowly but surely, your body is starting to understand that you're making the best decisions for your health. Start the day with a bright vegan mango lassi, inspired by traditional Indian flavors. Follow that with a protein-packed pad thai for lunch and a crisp bitter salad for dinner. For our exercises, we will train the abs, buttocks, back, and legs.

Mango Lassi

SERVES 2
PREP TIME: 5 minutes
PER SERVING: 167 calories, 2 g protein, 2 g fat, 30 g carbohydrates

1 mango
1¼ cups (300 ml) coconut milk
1 teaspoon ground cinnamon
3 ice cubes

1. Peel and pit the mango. Transfer to a blender with the rest of the ingredients and blend until smooth and creamy.

2. Pour into two glasses and serve.

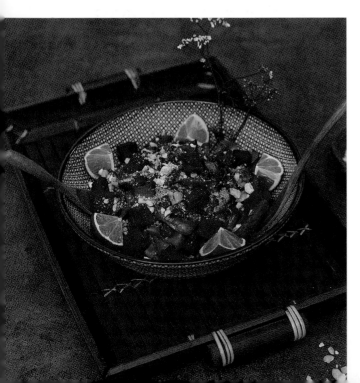

Pad Thai with Turmeric Tofu

SERVES 2
PREP TIME: 30 minutes
PER SERVING: 349 calories, 24 g protein, 20 g fat, 28 g carbohydrates

7 ounces (200 g) firm tofu
1 scallion
2 carrots
5 button mushrooms
1 teaspoon ground turmeric
1 tablespoon coconut oil
1 handful cilantro
1 lime
3½ ounces (100 g) wide rice noodles, cooked
1 handful cashews

SAUCE

⅓ cup (75 ml) soy sauce
1 to 2 tablespoons sriracha
1½ teaspoons maple syrup
1 tablespoon ground ginger

1. Drain the tofu, sandwich between several layers of kitchen towels to remove excess liquid, and dice.

2. Thinly slice the scallion, julienne the carrots, and quarter the mushrooms.

3. Toss the tofu with the turmeric until evenly coated. Heat the oil in a medium skillet over medium-high heat, add the tofu, and cook for 6 to 8 minutes until crispy. Set aside.

4. In a dry wok or large skillet over medium heat, sauté the scallion, carrots, and mushrooms until they begin to soften, about 7 minutes.

5. While the vegetables cook, make the sauce. Add all the ingredients to a small bowl and stir to combine.

6. Coarsely chop the cilantro, cut the lime into wedges, and set aside.

7. Pour the sauce into the wok with the vegetables and let everything simmer for 2 to 3 minutes, until the sauce has thickened slightly.

8. Fold in the tofu and the noodles, top with the cilantro, cashews, and lime wedges, and serve.

Radicchio and Hazelnut Salad

SERVES 2
PREP TIME: 20 minutes
PER SERVING: 409 calories, 6 g protein, 29 g fat, 29 g carbohydrates

¼ cup (40 g) peeled, blanched hazelnuts

1 head radicchio

2 pears

2 tablespoons watercress

DRESSING

3 tablespoons hazelnut oil

2 tablespoons balsamic vinegar

1 teaspoon Dijon mustard

1 tablespoon maple syrup

Sea salt

Fresh ground black pepper

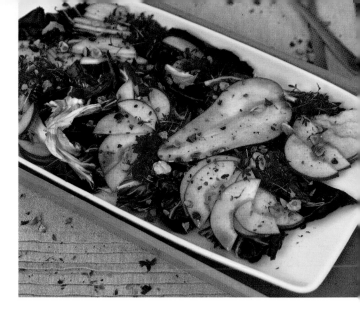

1. Coarsely chop the nuts and toast them in a dry skillet over medium heat for about 3 minutes, until fragrant.

2. Tear the radicchio into bite-size pieces onto a serving plate. Core and cut the pears into thin slices onto the radicchio.

3. To make the dressing, combine the oil, vinegar, mustard, and maple syrup in a small bowl. Season with salt and pepper.

4. Sprinkle the salad with the nuts and dressing and garnish with the watercress.

TODAY'S EXERCISES

EXERCISE 3:
Spinal Stretch + Sit-Up (page 68)

EXERCISE 4:
Quad Stretch + Knee Bend (page 70)

EXERCISE 7:
Calf Stretch + Lunge (page 76)

EXERCISE 10:
Full Body Stretch + Side Plank (page 82)

Today you have the privilege of trying out the best pudding in the world—and your body will thank you! If you're experiencing muscle pains today, that's OK: It's a sign that your muscles are slowly waking up from their deep sleep.

Raspberry Chia Pudding

SERVES 2
PREP TIME: 10 minutes
SOAKING TIME: 1 hour (or overnight)
PER SERVING: 229 calories, 8 g protein, 12 g fat, 12 g carbohydrates

1⅔ cups (400 ml) coconut milk

¼ cup (50 g) chia seeds

1 teaspoon ground cinnamon

7 ounces (200 g) raspberries

1 handful basil leaves

2 teaspoons shredded coconut

1. Stir the coconut milk, chia seeds, and cinnamon together in a small bowl. Pour the mixture into two glasses and put them in the refrigerator for at least 1 hour or overnight.

2. Blend the raspberries and basil in a blender until smooth. Pour over the chia puddings, sprinkle with the coconut, and serve.

Vegan Poke Bowls

SERVES 2
PREP TIME: 45 minutes
PER SERVING: 973 calories, 45 g protein, 31 g fat, 114 g carbohydrates

1 cup (200 g) brown rice

Sea salt

⅔ cups (100 g) edamame pods

1 avocado

1 mango

1 carrot

1 scallion

7 ounces (200 g) smoked tofu

1 tablespoon black sesame seeds

2 tablespoons soy sauce

1. Rinse the rice and prepare according to package instructions.

2. Bring a small pot of salted water to a boil, then add the edamame and let simmer for 7 minutes. Drain, rinse with cold water, and hull the beans.

3. Peel, pit, and slice the avocado and the mango. Julienne or spiralize the carrot. Cut the scallion into rings and the tofu into thin strips.

4. Place the cooked rice in the middle of a bowl and arrange the other ingredients nicely around it. Sprinkle with the sesame seeds and soy sauce and serve.

Quinoa and Spinach Salad with Cranberries

SERVES 2
PREP TIME: 25 minutes
PER SERVING: 277 calories, 10 g protein, 6 g fat, 41 g carbohydrates

½ cup (90 g) multicolored quinoa

½ cucumber

1 tablespoon chopped almonds

1 tablespoon dried cranberries

5 ounces (150 g) baby spinach

DRESSING

Juice of 1 orange

1 tablespoon olive oil

1 teaspoon mustard

Sea salt

Fresh ground black pepper

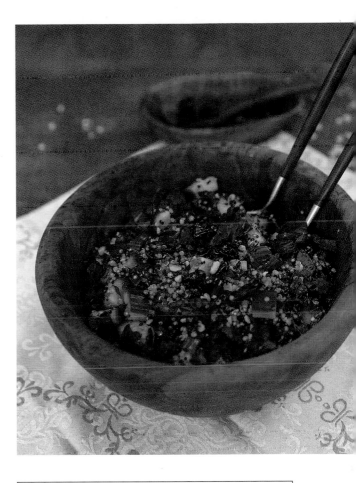

1. Pour the quinoa into a small pot with 1 cup (240 ml) water and bring to a boil. Reduce the heat to low and simmer until all the liquid has been absorbed, about 8 minutes. Set aside to cool.

2. Meanwhile, dice the cucumber and transfer to a bowl with the almonds and cranberries.

3. To make the dressing, mix the orange juice, oil, and mustard together in a small bowl. Season with salt and pepper and set aside.

4. Add the cooled quinoa to the cucumber, stir to combine, and pour on the dressing. Coarsely chop the spinach and fold into the salad. Divide between two bowls and serve.

TODAY'S EXERCISES

EXERCISE 5:
Hamstring Stretch + Diagonal Crunch with Leg Raise (page 72)

EXERCISE 6:
Chest Stretch + Superman (page 74)

EXERCISE 8:
Tricep Stretch + Push-Up (page 78)

EXERCISE 11:
Shoulder-Chest Stretch + Hip Dips (page 84)

Well rested and raring to go: Your biological clock is slowly getting used to your new rhythm and is rewarding you with increased secretion of melatonin, resulting in better sleep than ever.

Tropical Smoothie Bowl

SERVES 1
PREP TIME: 10 minutes
PER SERVING: 598 calories, 11 g protein, 8 g fat, 105 g carbohydrates

1 banana

1 mango

1⅓ cups (200 g) mixed berries (fresh or frozen)

Scant ½ cup (100 ml) orange juice

TOPPING

½ banana

1 tablespoon cacao nibs

1 tablespoon goji berries

1 tablespoon shredded coconut

1. Peel the banana, peel and pit the mango, and blend them together with the berries and the orange juice in a blender until smooth. Pour into a big bowl.

2. To make the topping, cut the banana into slices and arrange on top of the smoothie in the bowl. Sprinkle the cacao nibs, goji berries, and coconut in lines over the top, and serve.

Sweet Potato Coconut Curry

SERVES 2
PREP TIME: 25 minutes
PER SERVING: 378 calories, 5 g protein, 18 g fat, 46 g carbohydrates

1 large sweet potato (about 11 ounces/300 g)

1 carrot

1 red onion

1-inch (2.5 cm) piece ginger

1 garlic clove

1 tablespoon coconut oil

2 teaspoons curry powder

2 teaspoons ground turmeric

⅔ cup (150 ml) vegetable broth (see Note on page 174)

Scant ½ cup (100 ml) coconut milk

1 handful cilantro

12 cherry tomatoes, optional

Sea salt

Fresh ground black pepper

1. Peel and dice the sweet potato and the carrot. Peel and finely chop the onion, ginger, and garlic.

2. Heat the oil in a large saucepan over medium-high heat and add the onion, ginger, and garlic. Cook until fragrant, about 1 minute, then add the curry powder and turmeric. Stir in the sweet potato and carrot.

Add the broth and coconut milk and let simmer, uncovered, for 12 minutes, until the sauce has thickened.

3. Chop the cilantro and quarter the tomatoes, if using. Add to the pan and season with salt and pepper.

4. Divide between bowls and serve.

Parsley Salad with Amaranth

SERVES 2
PREP TIME: 15 minutes
PER SERVING: 350 calories, 10 g protein, 14 g fat, 40 g carbohydrates

2 bunches parsley

½ bunch mint

2 large beefsteak tomatoes

1 red onion

½ cup (90 g) puffed amaranth

DRESSING

Juice of 1 lemon

2 tablespoons olive oil

1 teaspoon ground cumin

Sea salt

Fresh ground black pepper

1. Roughly chop the herbs. Dice the tomatoes. Peel and dice the onion. Mix together in a bowl. Fold in the amaranth.

2. To make the dressing, mix the lemon juice, oil, and cumin in a small bowl and season with salt and pepper.

3. Pour the dressing over the salad and enjoy.

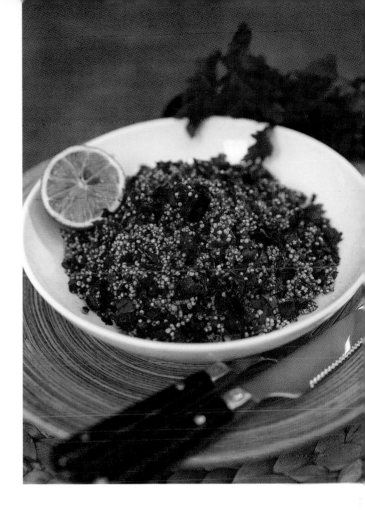

TODAY'S EXERCISES

EXERCISE 7:
Calf Stretch + Lunge (page 76)

EXERCISE 9:
Neck Stretch + Tabletop (page 80)

EXERCISE 10:
Full Body Stretch + Side Plank (page 82)

EXERCISE 12:
Rotation Stretches (page 86)

Congrats! You've made it to Day 5. Today's meal plan includes a delicious quinoa porridge, crispy fried eggplant, and a light tomato and melon salad. The exercises focus on your pelvis, spine, and shoulders. Keep going!

Quinoa-Berry Porridge

SERVES 2
PREP TIME: 25 minutes
PER SERVING: 186 calories, 6 g protein, 5 g fat, 28 g carbohydrates

---

⅓ cup (60 g) white quinoa

3 tablespoons almond milk (see page 145)

½ vanilla bean, scraped out, or 1½ teapoons vanilla extract

1 teaspoon ground cinnamon

1 tablespoon agave syrup

TOPPING

⅓ cup (50 g) frozen berries

1 tablespoon cacao nibs

1 teaspoon chopped almonds

---

1. Rinse the quinoa thoroughly with cold water. Transfer to a small pot with ¼ cup (60 ml) water, the almond milk, vanilla, and cinnamon and bring to a boil. Let the mixture simmer for 10 minutes, then sweeten with the agave syrup.

2. To make the topping, carefully warm the berries in a small pot.

3. Divide the porridge between two small bowls, pour the berries on top, and sprinkle with the cacao nibs and almonds.

Fried Eggplant with Capers

SERVES 2
PREP TIME: 30 minutes
PER SERVING: 168 calories, 7 g protein, 6 g fat, 16 g carbohydrates

---

2 medium eggplants

Sea salt

1 garlic clove

2 beefsteak tomatoes

3 tablespoons coconut oil

1 cup (100 g) dry-packed sun-dried tomatoes

2 tablespoons capers

Fresh ground black pepper

3 basil leaves

---

1. Dice the eggplants, sprinkle with salt, and let sit in a strainer for 30 minutes. Peel and finely chop the garlic and dice the beefsteak tomatoes. Set aside.

2. Pat the eggplant dry with a kitchen towel. Heat 2 tablespoons of the oil in a large skillet over medium-high heat. Add the eggplant and fry until crispy and golden, about 3 minutes. Set aside.

3. Heat the remaining oil in the skillet over medium heat. Add the diced tomatoes, garlic, and sun-dried tomatoes and simmer for 5 minutes.

4. Add the eggplant and capers and simmer for 10 more minutes, until any liquid has reduced.

5. Season with salt and pepper and garnish with the basil.

Tomato and Melon Salad

SERVES 2
PREP TIME: 20 minutes
PER SERVING: 542 calories, 15 g protein, 41 g fat, 25 g carbohydrates

1 pint mixed tomatoes (about 11 ounces/300 g)

1 red onion

Scant 1 cup (150 g) peeled, diced honeydew melon

1 handful mint

¾ cup (100 g) pine nuts

DRESSING

Juice of 1 lemon

1 tablespoon agave syrup

3 tablespoons olive oil

Sea salt

Fresh ground black pepper

1. Roughly chop the tomatoes. Peel the onion and slice into thin rings. Combine with the melon in a medium bowl. Roughly chop the mint and fold it into the salad.

2. Toast the pine nuts in a dry skillet over medium heat for 3 minutes, or until golden.

3. To make the dressing, mix the lemon juice, agave syrup, and oil in a small bowl, season with salt and pepper, then pour over the salad.

4. Top with the pine nuts and serve.

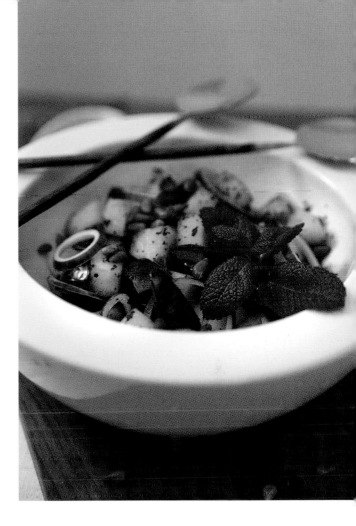

TODAY'S EXERCISES

EXERCISE 1:
Pelvis Down + Pelvis Up (page 64)

EXERCISE 3:
Spinal Stretch + Sit-Up (page 68)

EXERCISE 11:
Shoulder-Chest Stretch + Hip Dips (page 84)

EXERCISE 12:
Rotation Stretches (page 86)

Today's breakfast is an oatmeal, to attack superfluous cholesterol, with cinnamon to ensure a healthy blood sugar level. Lunch is a filling potato salad, and dinner keeps it light with a rainbow salad. You've almost made it through the week! These exercises announce to the body that things are looking up.

Apple-Cinnamon Overnight Oats

SERVES 2
PREP TIME: 10 minutes
SOAKING TIME: 8 hours (or overnight)
PER SERVING: 278 calories, 8 g protein, 7 g fat, 41 g carbohydrates

---

1 apple

1 cup (90 g) rolled oats

1 cup (240 ml) unsweetened almond milk (see page 145)

1 tablespoon goji berries

1 teaspoon ground cinnamon

10 hazelnuts

---

1. The night before, core and cut the apple in half. Coarsely grate one half and put the other half in the refrigerator. Mix the oats, grated apple, almond milk, goji berries, and cinnamon in a small bowl. Cover and let the mixture rest in the refrigerator overnight.

2. The next morning, coarsely chop the nuts and toast in a dry skillet over medium heat for about 3 minutes. Cut the second half of the apple into thin slices.

3. Stir the oat mixture, then divide between two bowls. Top with the apple slices and nuts and serve.

Potato Salad

SERVES 2
PREP TIME: 30 minutes
PER SERVING: 289 calories, 8 g protein, 1 g fat, 55 g carbohydrates

---

1¾ pounds (800 g) waxy potatoes

3 ounces (85 g) cornichons (about 17)

3 ounces (85 g) radishes (about 9 large)

1 handful dill

1 red onion

Sea salt

Fresh ground black pepper

DRESSING

¼ cup plus 2 tablespoons (90 ml) white vinegar

⅓ cup (80 ml) vegetable broth (see Note on page 174) or cornichon brine

2 tablespoons mustard

1 teaspoon maple syrup

---

1. Place the potatoes in a large pot and cover with cold water. Boil until fork tender, about 15 minutes. Let cool, peel, and cut into bite-size pieces.

2. Thinly slice the cornichons and radishes. Roughly chop the dill. Peel and dice the onion. Combine with the potatoes in a medium bowl.

3. To make the dressing, combine the vinegar and broth with the mustard and maple syrup in a small bowl until creamy.

4. Pour the dressing over the salad, mix, and season with salt and pepper. Divide between bowls and serve.

Rainbow Mason Jar Salad

SERVES 2
PREP TIME: 25 minutes
PER SERVING: 170 calories, 4 g protein, 7 g fat, 16 g carbohydrates

12 cherry tomatoes
4 mini bell peppers
4 handfuls baby spinach
2 handfuls blueberries
1 handful watercress

DRESSING

2 tablespoons balsamic vinegar
1 tablespoon olive oil
1 teaspoon Dijon mustard
1 teaspoon maple syrup
1 teaspoon sesame seeds
Sea salt
Fresh ground black pepper

1. Halve the tomatoes and slice the bell peppers.

2. To make the dressing, stir the vinegar, oil, mustard, maple syrup, and sesame seeds until creamy. Season with salt and pepper. Divide the dressing evenly between two jars.

3. Layer the vegetables in the jars: first the tomatoes, followed by the bell peppers, spinach, blueberries, and watercress. Cover and shake the jars to distribute the dressing evenly and serve.

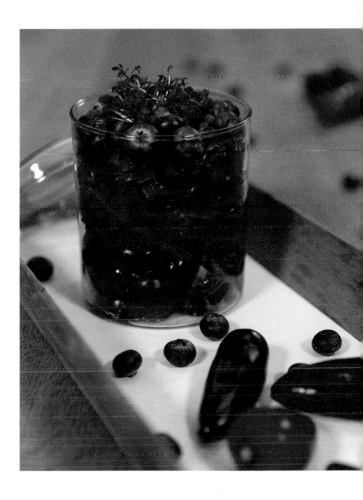

TODAY'S EXERCISES:

EXERCISE 2:
Hip Flexor Stretch + Bridge (page 66)

EXERCISE 4:
Quad Stretch + Knee Bend (page 70)

EXERCISE 5:
Hamstring Stretch + Diagonal Crunch with Leg Raise (page 72)

EXERCISE 6:
Chest Stretch + Superman (page 74)

DAY 7

You made it through the first week of intermittent fasting! It's halftime and your day off from exercises. Now is the time to enjoy things: meditate, read a book, go to the spa, or just be lazy. You earned it!

Rainbow Fruit Salad

SERVES 2
PREP TIME: 15 minutes
PER SERVING: 253 calories, 3 g protein, 2 g fat, 49 g carbohydrates

1 apple
1⅓ cups (200 g) strawberries
1⅓ cups (200 g) grapes
1 banana
⅔ cup (100 g) blueberries
1 handful mint leaves
Juice of 1 lime
1 teaspoon ground cinnamon

1. Dice the apple and strawberries, halve the grapes, and peel and slice the banana. Combine with the blueberries in a medium bowl.

2. Chop the mint and fold into the salad. Pour in the lime juice and mix.

3. Divide the salad between two bowls, sprinkle with the cinnamon, and serve.

Wild Rice and Fennel Stir-Fry

SERVES 2
PREP TIME: 30 minutes
PER SERVING: 345 calories, 8 g protein, 11 g fat, 49 g carbohydrates

⅔ cup (100 g) mixed wild and brown rice
1 cup (240 ml) vegetable broth (see Note on page 174)
1 red onion
1 garlic clove
2 fennel bulbs, with fronds
2 tablespoons canola oil
3 tablespoons white balsamic vinegar
Sea salt
Fresh ground black pepper

1. Bring the rice and broth to a boil in a small pot, then reduce the heat to low and simmer for 20 minutes, or until the rice is tender and the broth has been absorbed.

2. Peel and dice the onion and peel and mince the garlic. Chop the fennel fronds and set them aside. Cut the fennel bulbs in half and then into slices.

3. Heat the oil in a medium skillet over medium heat and fry the onion and garlic for 2 minutes. Add the fennel bulb and cook for 12 minutes, or until the fennel has softened. Deglaze with the vinegar and season with salt and pepper.

4. Arrange the fennel and rice on a plate, sprinkle with the chopped fennel fronds, and serve.

Fresh Cucumber and Radish Salad

SERVES 2
PREP TIME: 25 minutes
PER SERVING: 70 calories, 1 g protein, 1 g fat, 13 g carbohydrates

1 cucumber

8 radishes

½ red onion

½ bunch dill

Sea salt

Fresh ground black pepper

DRESSING

2 tablespoons white balsamic vinegar

1 tablespoon agave syrup

Juice of 1 lemon

1. Chop the cucumber. Remove the radish greens, then quarter the radishes. Peel and dice the onion, and roughly chop the dill. Combine in a medium bowl.

2. To make the dressing, mix the vinegar with the agave syrup and lemon juice.

3. Pour the dressing over the salad. Season with salt and pepper and serve.

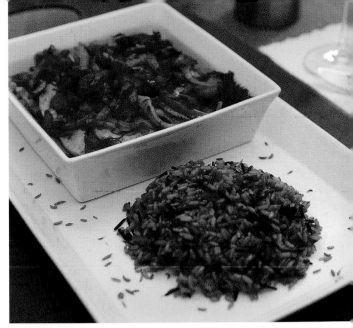

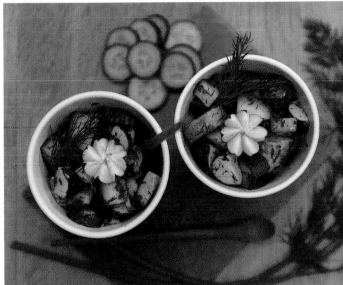

TODAY'S EXERCISES

As mentioned, today is your day off! Use this time to go outdoors, get some fresh air, and relax. Maybe you'd like to take a long walk or just lie around on your couch. Enjoy the success of having completed the first week of fasting.

Doesn't it feel great to have made it through a whole week? By now, your new routine should be getting easier and easier. Have fun with your second week of intermittent fasting with all new recipes and workout plans.

Avocado-Berry Bowl

SERVES 2
PREP TIME: 10 minutes
PER SERVING: 392 calories, 5 g protein, 20 g fat, 42 g carbohydrates

1 avocado

1 pear

1 apple

1 banana

1 handful blackberries

1 handful blueberries

¼ cup (60 ml) lime juice

2 tablespoons pomegranate seeds

2 tablespoons walnuts

1. Cut the avocado in half, remove the pit, and dice the flesh. Core and dice the pear and the apple. Peel and slice the banana. Combine in a medium bowl with the blackberries and blueberries.

2. Pour in the lime juice and mix. Top with the pomegranate seeds and walnuts and serve.

Glass Noodle Salad

SERVES 2
PREP TIME: 20 minutes
PER SERVING: 415 calories, 11 g protein, 14 g fat, 56 g carbohydrates

3½ ounces (100 g) glass noodles (bean thread vermicelli)

1 scallion

1 carrot

4 mini bell peppers

1 bunch cilantro

1 handful broccoli florets

1 handful cashews

DRESSING

2 tablespoons soy sauce

2 tablespoons rice vinegar

Juice of 1 lemon

3 tablespoons sesame seeds

Sea salt

Fresh ground black pepper

1. Soak the noodles in hot water for 5 minutes. Rinse under cold water, drain, and set aside.

2. Thinly slice the scallion and julienne the carrot and bell peppers. Roughly chop the cilantro. Combine with the noodles and broccoli in a large bowl and mix well.

3. To make the dressing, mix the soy sauce, rice vinegar, and lemon juice in a small bowl and add the sesame seeds. Season with salt and pepper.

4. Pour the dressing over the salad, mix, and let sit for 7 minutes. Divide between bowls, garnish with the cashews, and serve.

Broccoli and Zucchini Stir-Fry

SERVES 2
PREP TIME: 20 minutes
PER SERVING: 280 calories, 10 g protein, 21 g fat, 9 g carbohydrates

1 head broccoli

1 zucchini

3 tablespoons sliced almonds

1 red onion

1 garlic clove

1 tablespoon coconut oil

Scant ½ cup (100 ml) coconut milk

1 teaspoon dried thyme

1 teaspoon dried oregano

Sea salt

Fresh ground black pepper

1. Cut the broccoli into small pieces. Cut the zucchini in half and then into thin slices. Toast the sliced almonds in a small dry skillet over medium heat until golden, about 3 minutes.

2. Peel and dice the onion and peel and mince the garlic. Heat the oil in a skillet and fry until softened, about 5 minutes.

3. Add the broccoli and zucchini and cook for 2 minutes, then add the coconut milk.

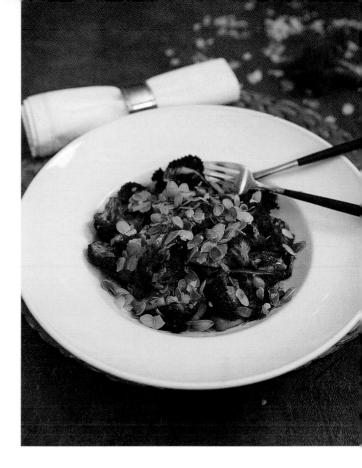

4. Add the thyme and oregano and season with salt and pepper. Garnish with the almonds and serve.

TODAY'S EXERCISES

EXERCISE 1:
Pelvis Down + Pelvis Up (page 64)

EXERCISE 5:
Hamstring Stretch + Diagonal Crunch with Leg Raise (page 72)

EXERCISE 8:
Tricep Stretch + Push-Up (page 78)

EXERCISE 10:
Full Body Stretch + Side Plank (page 82)

DAY 9

Did you know that beets can help regulate your blood pressure? Today's exercises are relaxing and calming, ensuring that you breathe deeply, and that your blood pressure is normalized.

Red Power Smoothie

SERVES 2
PREP TIME: 10 minutes
PER SERVING: 147 calories, 3 g protein, 1 g fat, 22 g carbohydrates

2 medium beets

1 lemon

1 banana

1-inch (2.5 cm) piece ginger

1⅓ cups (200 g) mixed berries

1¼ cups (300 ml) coconut water

1 handful mint leaves

1. Peel and chop the beets. Peel and slice the lemon and the banana. Peel and finely chop the ginger.

2. Add all of the ingredients to a blender, reserving a few mint leaves. Blend until smooth and creamy.

3. Divide the smoothie between two glasses, garnish with the reserved mint leaves, and serve.

Chickpea and Spinach Curry

SERVES 2
PREP TIME: 20 minutes
PER SERVING: 643 calories, 26 g protein, 38 g fat, 27 g carbohydrates

1 pound 5 ounces (600 g) baby spinach

1 yellow onion

1-inch (2.5 cm) piece ginger

2 garlic cloves

2 tablespoons coconut oil

1 teaspoon garam masala

1 cup (240 ml) coconut milk

1 cup (200 g) drained, rinsed canned chickpeas

1 teaspoon ground cumin

Sea salt

Fresh ground black pepper

4 popadams (thin lentil flatbreads), optional

1. Julienne the spinach. Peel and finely dice the onion, ginger, and garlic.

2. Heat the oil in a large skillet over medium heat, then add the onion, garlic, and ginger. Cook for 5 minutes, stirring constantly, until softened.

3. Add the garam masala and spinach and cook for 1 minute, then add the coconut milk, chickpeas, and cumin and simmer for a few minutes, until the desired consistency is reached. Season with salt and pepper and serve with the popadams, if using.

Beet and Radicchio Carpaccio

SERVES 2
PREP TIME: 20 minutes
PER SERVING: 360 calories, 13 g protein,
12 g fat, 44 g carbohydrates

¼ cup (50 g) beluga lentils

4 beets

2 heads radicchio

¼ cup (40 g) pomegranate seeds

1 handful mixed berries

DRESSING

¼ cup (60 ml) lemon juice

3 tablespoons balsamic vinegar

2 tablespoons extra virgin olive oil

1 teaspoon dried thyme

Sea salt

Fresh ground black pepper

1. Cook the lentils according to package instructions, then drain and let cool.

2. While the lentils cook, peel and cut the beets into thin slices with a sharp knife or mandoline. Wash the radicchio and separate the leaves. Arrange the beets and radicchio on a serving plate.

3. To make the dressing, combine the lemon juice, vinegar, oil, and thyme in a small bowl. Season with salt and pepper.

4. Toss the salad with the dressing, then top with the lentils, pomegranate seeds, and berries, and serve.

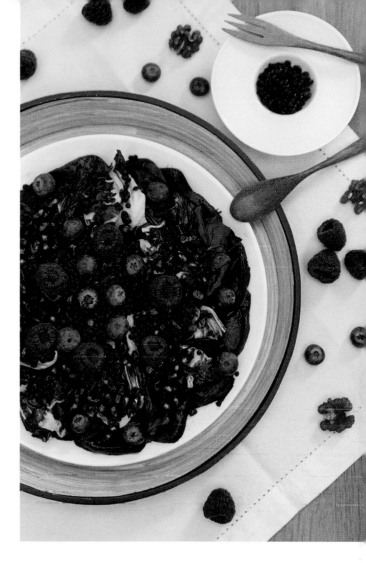

TODAY'S EXERCISES

EXERCISE 2:
Hip Flexor Stretch + Bridge (page 66)

EXERCISE 6:
Chest Stretch + Superman (page 74)

EXERCISE 9:
Neck Stretch + Tabletop (page 80)

EXERCISE 12:
Rotation Stretches (page 86)

Congratulations! By today you can be sure that every cell in your body has shifted into health mode. So, keep at it: Enjoy your meals and stick with those exercises!

Coconut Millet Porridge

SERVES 2
PREP TIME: 10 minutes
PER SERVING: 200 calories, 5 g protein, 3 g fat, 36 g carbohydrates

1¼ cups (300 ml) coconut milk

1 teaspoon ground cinnamon

1 cup (80 g) millet

½ orange

1 tablespoon pomegranate seeds

1. Combine the coconut milk and cinnamon with 1¼ cups (300 ml) water in a small pot over high heat. Add the millet and bring to a boil. Turn the heat to low and simmer for 8 minutes, or until the water has absorbed. Remove from the heat and set aside.

2. While the millet cooks, peel and slice the orange.

3. Divide the porridge between two bowls, garnish with the orange slices and pomegranate seeds, and serve.

Zucchini Noodles with Tofu and Avocado

SERVES 2
PREP TIME: 25 minutes
PER SERVING: 521 calories, 23 g protein, 39 g fat, 14 g carbohydrates

7 ounces (200 g) smoked tofu

2 zucchini

1 garlic clove

6 cherry tomatoes

1 avocado

2 tablespoons olive oil

Sea salt

Fresh ground black pepper

Juice of 1 lemon

4 basil sprigs

1. Dice the tofu. Cut the ends off the zucchini, then, using a spiralizer or vegetable peeler, cut the zucchini into thin noodles. Peel and thinly slice the garlic. Halve the tomatoes. Cut the avocado in half, remove the pit, and peel and dice the flesh.

2. Heat the oil in a medium skillet over medium heat, then add the garlic and sauté for 1 minute, until fragrant.

3. Add the tofu, followed by the tomatoes. Sauté for 2 minutes, stirring frequently. Remove from the heat and season with salt and pepper.

4. Transfer the zucchini noodles to a large bowl, then add the tofu mixture and avocado. Sprinkle with lemon juice and stir to combine. Season again with salt and pepper, garnish with the basil, and serve.

Spanish Tomato Salad

SERVES 2
PREP TIME: 25 minutes
PER SERVING: 264 calories, 6 g protein, 16 g fat, 17 g carbohydrates

4 beefsteak tomatoes

½ red onion

1 banana pepper

½ bunch basil

SALSA

1 beefsteak tomato

½ red onion

1 garlic clove

3 tablespoons olive oil

2 tablespoons apple cider vinegar

½ bunch basil

Sea salt

Fresh ground black pepper

1. Roughly chop the tomatoes. Peel and finely dice the onion. Cut the pepper into rings and roughly chop most of the basil, setting aside some pepper rings and basil leaves for garnish. Transfer the rest of the vegetables to a medium bowl and stir to combine.

2. To make the salsa, roughly chop the tomato, peel and chop the onion and garlic, then add to a blender with the oil, vinegar, and basil. Blend until smooth, season with salt and pepper, and pour over the salad.

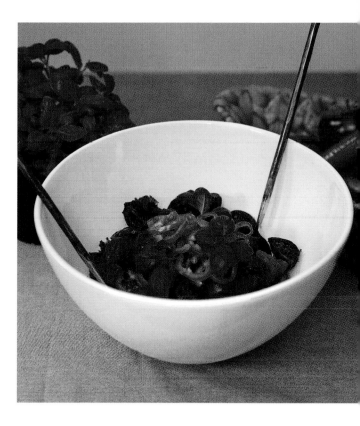

3. Garnish with the reserved pepper rings and basil leaves and serve.

TODAY'S EXERCISES

EXERCISE 1:
Pelvis Down + Pelvis Up (page 64)

EXERCISE 4:
Quad Stretch + Knee Bend (page 70)

EXERCISE 7:
Calf Stretch + Lunge (page 76)

EXERCISE 11:
Shoulder-Chest Stretch + Hip Dips (page 84)

Today, let's do something good for your immune system and give it loads of antioxidants. Hopefully, you're seeing improvements in your mood every day. And you're probably feeling better and more energetic than you were before!

Berry Chia Bowl

SERVES 1
PREP TIME: 10 minutes
SOAKING TIME: 1 hour (or overnight)
PER SERVING: 489 calories, 12 g protein, 19 g fat, 55 g carbohydrates

3 tablespoons chia seeds
⅔ cup (150 ml) coconut milk
1 banana
1 cup (150 g) fresh mixed berries
Scant ½ cup (100 ml) unsweetened cranberry juice

TOPPING
½ pear
1 tablespoon walnuts
⅓ cup (50 g) fresh mixed berries

1. Combine the chia seeds and coconut milk in a small bowl and put in the refrigerator to soak for at least 1 hour.

2. Remove the chia pudding from the fridge and transfer to a blender. Peel the banana and add it to the blender along with the berries and juice. Blend until smooth and creamy, then transfer to a bowl.

3. To top, slice the pear and roughly chop the walnuts. Sprinkle over the bowl with the berries and serve.

Citrusy Squash Salad

SERVES 2
PREP TIME: 20 minutes
PER SERVING: 246 calories, 3 g protein, 20 g fat, 11 g carbohydrates

½ red kuri or ¼ butternut squash
3 tablespoons olive oil
1 teaspoon fennel seeds
Sea salt
Fresh ground black pepper
4 unpeeled garlic cloves
2 handfuls watercress

DRESSING
Juice of 1 lemon
3 tablespoons coconut cream
1 tablespoon fennel seeds
2 teaspoons Dijon mustard
Sea salt
Fresh ground black pepper

1. Preheat the oven to 350°F (180°C). Line a baking sheet with parchment paper.

2. Cut the squash into slices about 1 inch (2.5 cm) thick. Transfer to a medium bowl. Add the oil and fennel seeds, season with salt and pepper, and mix well. Transfer along with the garlic to the baking sheet and roast for 15 minutes, or until tender.

3. While the squash cooks, make the dressing. In a small bowl, mix the lemon juice with the coconut cream, fennel seeds, and mustard until it becomes a creamy sauce. Season with salt and pepper.

4. Remove the squash from the oven and arrange on a serving plate with the watercress. Toss with the dressing and serve.

Smoked Tofu and Lentil Stew

SERVES 2
PREP TIME: 30 minutes
PER SERVING: 584 calories, 39 g protein, 12 g fat, 68 g carbohydrates

1 red onion

½ leek

2 carrots

4 medium potatoes

½ parsley root or celery root

2 tablespoons vegetable oil

1⅔ cups (400 ml) vegetable broth (see Note on page 174)

¾ cup (150 g) brown lentils

1 teaspoon dried thyme

1 teaspoon dried marjoram

7 ounces (200 g) smoked tofu

Sea salt

Fresh ground black pepper

1. Peel and finely dice the onion. Wash the leek and cut into thin rings. Peel the carrots, potatoes, and parsley root and dice them.

2. Warm the oil in a large pot over medium-high heat, then add the onion and leek and sauté until slightly softened, about 3 minutes. Stir in the carrots, potatoes, and parsley root and sauté for another 3 minutes. Deglaze with the broth, scraping the bottom of the pot.

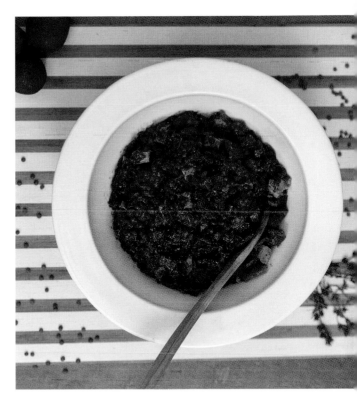

3. Add the lentils, thyme, and marjoram and simmer for 20 minutes. Dice the tofu, then add it to the stew, and stir until the tofu is warmed through. Season with salt and pepper, divide between bowls, and serve.

TODAY'S EXERCISES

EXERCISE 2:
Hip Flexor Stretch + Bridge (page 66)

EXERCISE 3:
Spinal Stretch + Sit-Up (page 68)

EXERCISE 6:
Chest Stretch + Superman (page 74)

EXERCISE 9:
Neck Stretch + Tabletop (page 80)

By now you know exactly what it means to be full of energy. Your body has cleaned house and you should be feeling better than ever! Keep it up by starting your day with an energizing smoothie and working your whole body with these strengthening exercises.

Energy Smoothie

SERVES 2
PREP TIME: 10 minutes
PER SERVING: 133 calories, 2 g protein, 1 g fat, 23 g carbohydrates

1 apple

1 kiwi

¼ pineapple

½ cucumber

½ bunch parsley

1 cup (240 ml) coconut water

1 handful ice cubes

1. Core the apple, peel the kiwi and the pineapple, then roughly chop and transfer to a blender.

2. Add the cucumber, parsley, coconut water, and ice. Blend until creamy, then pour into two glasses and serve.

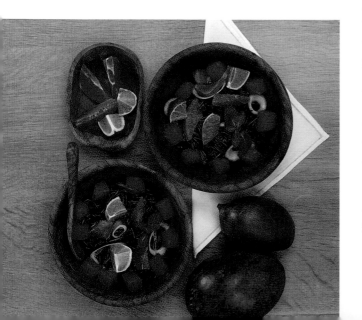

Black Rice with Mint and Citrus

SERVES 2
PREP TIME: 25 minutes
PER SERVING: 703 calories, 13 g protein, 15 g fat, 119 g carbohydrates

1 cup (200 g) black rice

1 mango

2 oranges

1 bunch fresh mint

1 red onion

Sea salt

Fresh ground black pepper

2 limes

DRESSING

2 tablespoons olive oil

2 tablespoons soy sauce

Juice of 1 orange

2 teaspoons Dijon mustard

1. Cook the rice according to the package instructions, drain, and let sit.

2. Peel, pit, and dice the mango. Peel and cut the oranges into sections. Roughly chop the mint. Peel the onion and cut into thin rings. Top the rice with the oranges and mango in a medium bowl. Add the mint and season with salt and pepper.

3. To make the dressing, mix all the ingredients together in a small bowl.

4. Pour the dressing over the salad and stir to combine. Cut the limes into wedges and serve alongside the salad.

Colorful Minestrone

SERVES 2
PREP TIME: 30 minutes
PER SERVING: 198 calories, 7 g protein, 6 g fat, 23 g carbohydrates

1 zucchini

1 carrot

2 bell peppers

1 scallion

½ celery root

⅔ cup (100 g) peeled, diced potato

1 tablespoon coconut oil

4 cups (1 L) vegetable broth (see Note on page 174)

1 handful parsley

Sea salt

Fresh ground black pepper

1. Dice the zucchini and carrot. Core, seed, and dice the peppers. Thinly slice the scallion. Peel and dice the celery root.

2. Heat the oil in a large pot, then add the vegetables and sauté for 3 minutes. Deglaze with the broth and simmer for 20 minutes. Remove from the heat.

3. Chop the parsley, then add to the pot. Season with salt and pepper and serve.

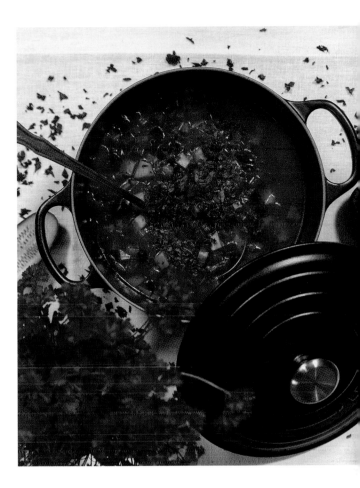

<table>
<tr><td colspan="1" align="center">TODAY'S EXERCISES</td></tr>
</table>

TODAY'S EXERCISES

EXERCISE 4:
Quad Stretch + Knee Bend (page 70)

EXERCISE 5:
Hamstring Stretch + Diagonal Crunch with Leg Raise (page 72)

EXERCISE 7:
Calf Stretch + Lunge (page 76)

EXERCISE 12:
Rotation Stretches (page 86)

Today is detox day! It's a good opportunity to take some time for self-care. Spend some time in the sauna or get a massage. You're worth it.

Strawberry Overnight Oats

SERVES 2
PREP TIME: 5 minutes
SOAKING TIME: 8 hours (or overnight)
PER SERVING: 238 calories, 8 g protein, 8 g fat, 28 g carbohydrates

---

1 cup (90 g) rolled oats

1 teaspoon chia seeds

1 teaspoon flaxseeds

1 teaspoon ground cinnamon

1 cup (240 ml) almond milk (see page 145)

1 handful strawberries, hulled and sliced

1 tablespoon chopped almonds

---

1. The night before, mix the oats, chia seeds, flaxseeds, cinnamon, and almond milk in a medium bowl. Cover and place in the refrigerator for at least 8 hours or overnight.

2. The following morning, remove the oats from the refrigerator, stir thoroughly, and divide between two bowls. Top with the strawberries and almonds and serve.

Potato Soup

SERVES 2
PREP TIME: 25 minutes
PER SERVING: 185 calories, 6 g protein, 1 g fat, 35 g carbohydrates

---

1 pound (450 g) Yukon Gold potatoes

1 large carrot

1 small celery root

1 small leek

1 bunch parsley

2½ cups (600 ml) vegetable broth (see Note on page 174)

Sea salt

Fresh ground black pepper

1 teaspoon ground nutmeg

---

1. Peel and dice the potatoes, carrot, and celery root. Wash and slice the leek. Chop the parsley.

2. Pour the broth into a large pot and add the vegetables. Bring to a boil and turn the heat to low to simmer for 15 minutes. Add half of the parsley and blend the soup with an immersion blender, leaving a few potato chunks intact if desired.

3. Season with salt and pepper. Sprinkle on the nutmeg and the rest of the parsley, then divide between bowls and serve.

Sauerkraut and Pear Salad with Smoked Tofu

SERVES 2
PREP TIME: 25 minutes
PER SERVING: 570 calories, 22 g protein, 35 g fat, 37 g carbohydrates

7 ounces (200 g) smoked tofu

1 tablespoon vegetable oil

2 pears

1⅓ cups (200 g) drained sauerkraut

3 tablespoons chopped almonds

2 figs, quartered

DRESSING

3 tablespoons apple juice

3 tablespoons olive oil

2 tablespoons apple cider vinegar

1 tablespoon agave syrup

Sea salt

Fresh ground black pepper

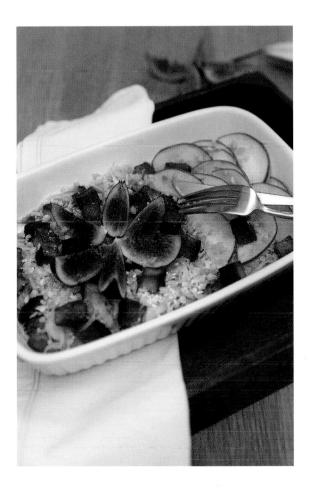

1. Cube the tofu. Heat the oil in a medium skillet and fry the tofu until crispy, about 6 minutes. Thinly slice the pears and transfer to a serving bowl with the sauerkraut and tofu.

2. To make the dressing, mix the apple juice, oil, vinegar, and agave syrup in a small bowl, then season with salt and pepper.

3. Pour the dressing over the salad and stir to combine. Top with the almonds and figs and serve.

TODAY'S EXERCISES

EXERCISE 3:
Spinal Stretch + Sit-Up (page 68)

EXERCISE 6:
Chest Stretch + Superman (page 74)

EXERCISE 8:
Tricep Stretch + Push-Up (page 78)

EXERCISE 11:
Shoulder-Chest Stretch + Hip Dips (page 84)

DAY 14

Congratulations! You've reached the end of the 14-Day Program, and now it's time to celebrate. Want to meet up with some friends? Just scale the recipes up for your guests. Maybe your success can convince them to try intermittent fasting, too. Take a day off from the exercises and enjoy allowing your body the time to clean up and close the construction sites.

Banana-Chocolate Chia Pudding

SERVES 2
PREP TIME: 10 minutes
SOAKING TIME: 1 hour (or overnight)
PER SERVING: 341 calories, 10 g protein, 15 g fat, 34 carbohydrates

¼ cup plus 2 tablespoons (70 g) chia seeds

1 tablespoon raw cacao powder

1¼ cups (300 ml) rice milk

TOPPING

1 banana

3½ tablespoons (50 ml) rice milk

2 tablespoons cacao nibs

1. Combine the chia seeds with the cacao powder and rice milk in a medium bowl, then divide between two glasses, cover, and refrigerate for at least 1 hour or overnight.

2. To make the topping, blend the banana and rice milk in a blender until smooth and creamy.

3. Pour the banana mixture over the pudding, sprinkle with the cacao nibs, and serve.

Avocado and Mango Salad

SERVES 2
PREP TIME: 20 minutes
PER SERVING: 325 calories, 4 g protein, 18 g fat, 30 g carbohydrates

1 avocado

1 cucumber

1 mango

1 bunch cilantro

Juice of 1 lemon

1 tablespoon olive oil

1 teaspoon cayenne pepper, or to taste

Sea salt

1. Peel, pit, and dice the avocado. Slice the cucumber. Peel and pit the mango. Slice part of the mango and dice the rest. Transfer the avocado, cucumber, and diced mango to a medium bowl and stir to combine. Roughly chop and fold in the cilantro.

2. Mix in the lemon juice, oil, and cayenne. Season with salt, top with the mango slices, then serve.

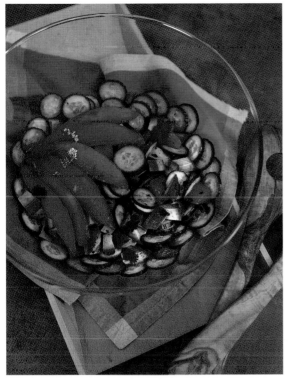

Carrot-Ginger Soup

SERVES 2
PREP TIME: 20 minutes
PER SERVING: 336 calories, 4 g protein,
28 g fat, 16 g carbohydrates

1 small red onion

1-inch (2.5 cm) piece ginger

3 cups (400 g) diced carrots

1 tablespoon coconut oil

1 cup (240 ml) coconut milk

1⅔ cups (400 ml) vegetable broth (see
  Note on page 174)

Sea salt

Fresh ground black pepper

Pumpkin seeds

Pomegranate seeds

1. Peel and dice the onion and ginger. Heat the oil in a large pot over medium-high heat, then add the onion and sauté until translucent, about 5 minutes. Add the ginger and carrots and sauté for 2 minutes more, until slightly softened.

2. Pour in the coconut milk, scraping up any bits at the bottom of the pot. Add the broth, bring to a boil, then turn the heat to low and simmer for 15 minutes. Puree with an immersion blender until smooth.

3. Season with salt and pepper. Top with the pumpkin and pomegranate seeds and serve.

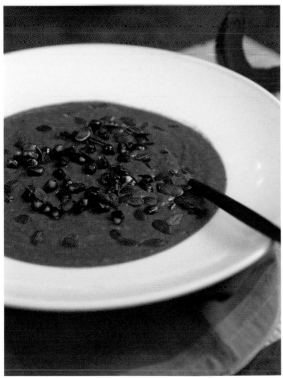

TODAY'S EXERCISES

Take some deep breaths and
enjoy your success!

Stick with It

Over the course of the past fourteen days, many big changes have taken place in your body. Above all, you have laid the foundation for a healthy lifestyle. Fourteen days of a purely plant-based diet have initiated processes that will only gain momentum going forward—toward complete cell rejuvenation. You just have to stick with it!

The best thing to do now is just to keep up this routine. Use the recipes on the following pages to continue. If the past fourteen days were extremely difficult for you, modify the program so that you can still enjoy your life. If it meant tormenting yourself because you missed eating meat and sweets, then go ahead and eat some, in moderation. Try as best you can to keep your diet 95 percent vegan and mostly sugar-free.

Don't despair if you go overboard once in a while—that's what cheat days are for! What's important is the long-term goal on your horizon. And keep moving, as much as possible. You can do it!

PART THREE

75 Delicious Vegan Recipes for Life

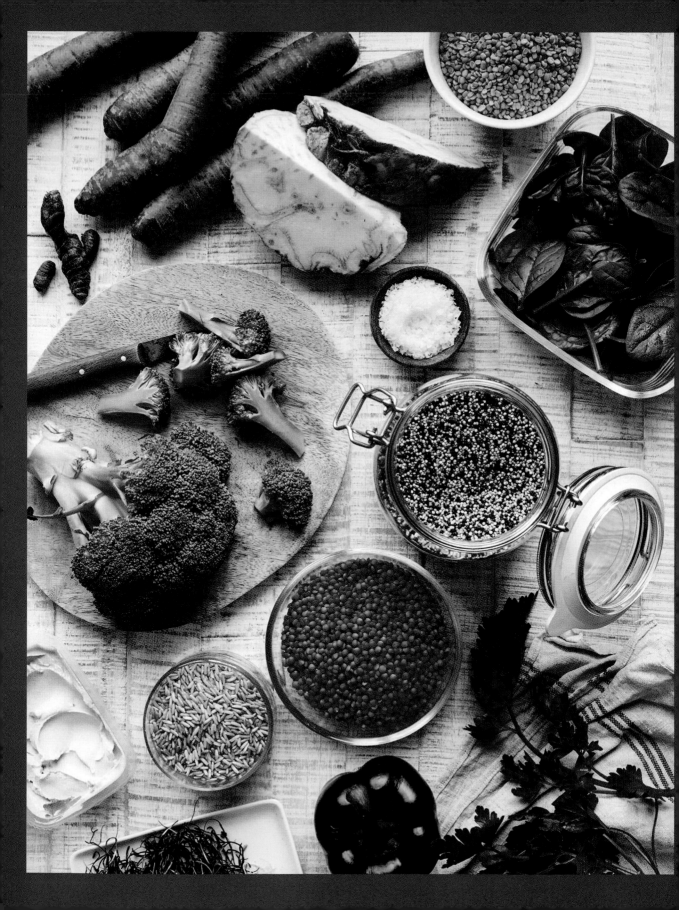

After you've completed the 14-Day Program, you'll need some more recipes to add to your repertoire. This section includes many more recipes that show how a healthy diet need be neither boring nor dull. Everything is so tasty that you'll look forward to your next meal, and so varied that your body gets exactly what it needs at any given moment. Then you will be both fit *and* healthy. Have fun cooking!

The Meals

The recipes are divided up into four chapters:

- From page 138 on you will find recipes for the first meal of the day, which should consist largely of fresh, easily digestible foods—the perfect start to a new day.

- The second meal of the day should contain healthy carbohydrates. They guarantee that your body gets the proper energy boost it needs. These recipes start on page 160.

- The third and final meal of the day (see page 212) provides your body with valuable proteins and prepares it to do its regeneration work during the sixteen-hour fasting phase.

- If you want to treat yourself to some sweets, head to page 250, where we have provided some recipes that prove that sweet treats can still be healthy and good for you.

Breakfast

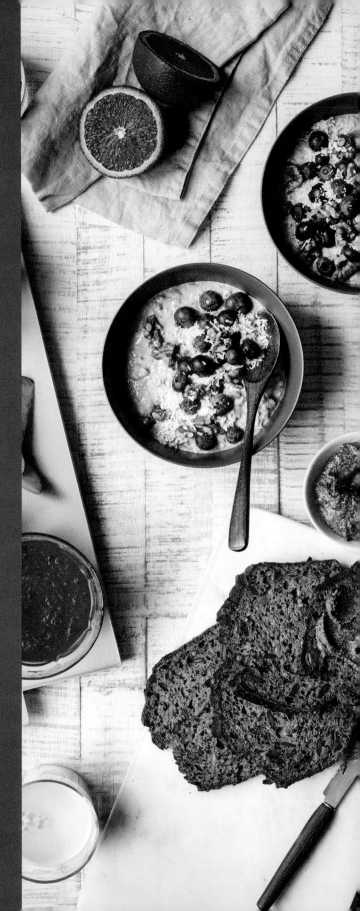

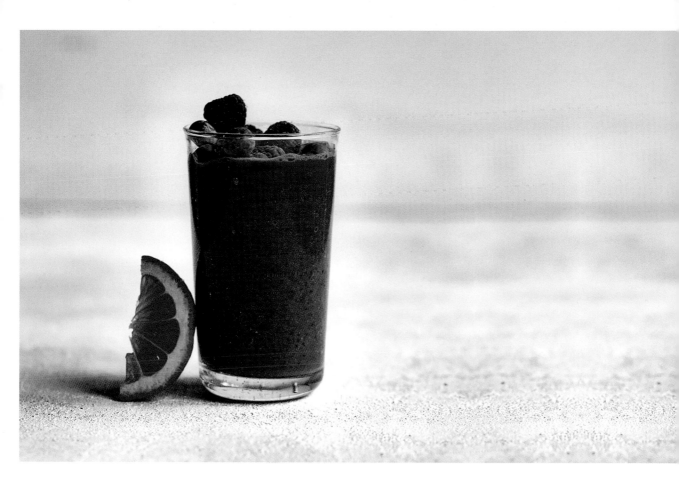

Avocado-Chard Smoothie

SERVES 1
PREP TIME: 10 minutes
PER SERVING: 500 calories, 5 g protein,
46 g fat, 17 g carbohydrates

3 chard leaves

1 avocado

1 handful fresh raspberries, strawberries,
  or blueberries

1 Medjool date, pitted

Juice of 1 lemon

Scant ½ cup (100 ml) coconut water

1. Tear the chard leaves into bite-size
pieces. Cut the avocado in half, remove the
pit, and scoop out the flesh with a spoon.
Transfer to a blender.

2. Add the remaining ingredients and
blend until creamy. Pour into a glass, top
with additional berries, if desired, and
enjoy.

Kale-Apple Smoothie

SERVES 1
PREP TIME: 10 minutes
PER SERVING: 130 calories, 3 g protein,
1 g fat, 3 g carbohydrates

3 kale leaves
1 apple
1 orange
1-inch (2.5 cm) piece ginger

1. Roughly chop the kale and core and dice the apple. Peel the orange and the ginger. Slice the orange and roughly chop the ginger.

2. Transfer to a blender with ⅔ cup (160 ml) water and blend until creamy. Pour into a glass and enjoy.

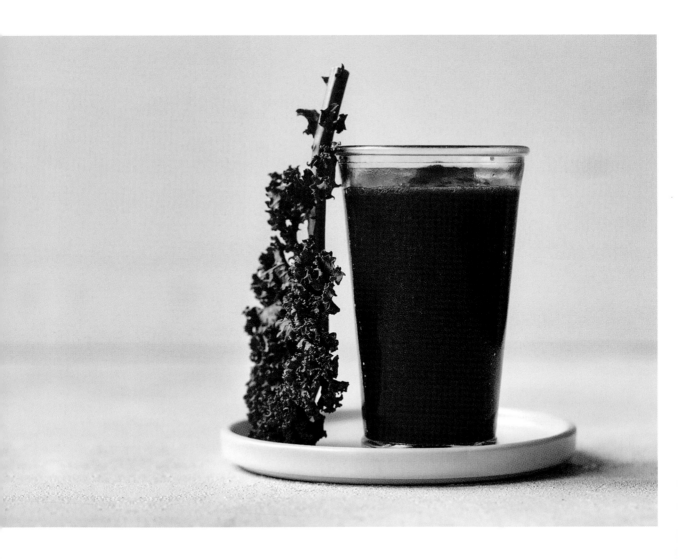

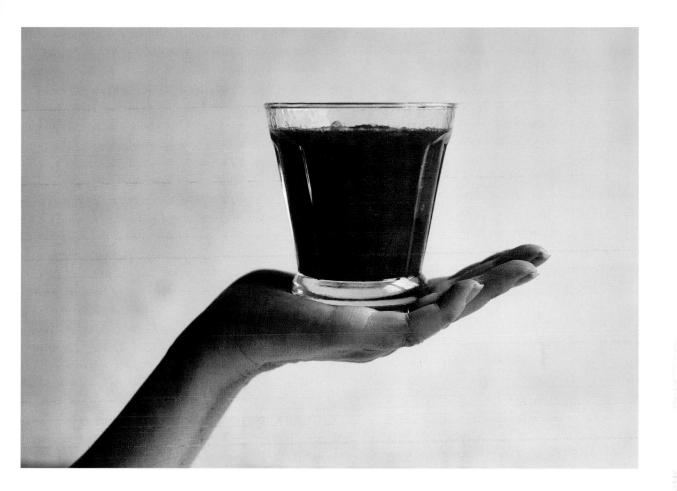

Carrot-Apple Smoothie

SERVES 2
PREP TIME: 10 minutes
PER SERVING: 120 calories, 1 g protein,
6 g fat, 15 g carbohydrates

---

1 large carrot
1 apple
1 orange
1-inch (2.5 cm) piece ginger
Juice of 1 lemon
1 tablespoon flaxseed oil
4 ice cubes

---

1. Dice the carrot. Quarter and core the apple. Peel and slice the orange. Peel and coarsely chop the ginger.

2. Transfer to a blender with the remaining ingredients and blend until creamy. Divide between glasses and enjoy.

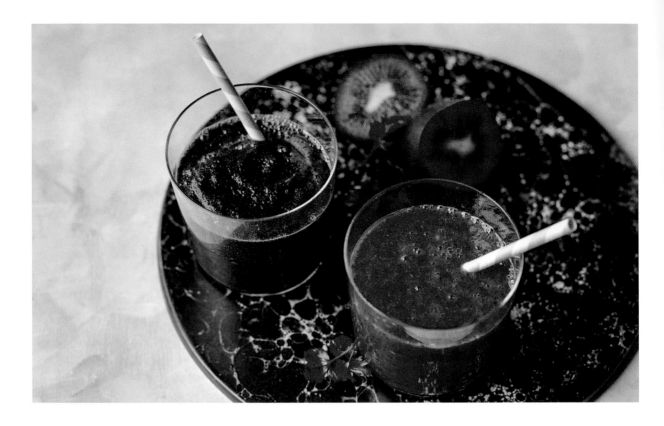

Beet-Carrot Smoothie

SERVES 1
PREP TIME: 10 minutes
PER SERVING: 150 calories, 4 g protein,
1 g fat, 30 g carbohydrates

1 beet
1 large carrot
1 orange
1-inch (2.5 cm) piece ginger
2 Medjool dates, pitted

1. Dice the beet and carrot. Peel and slice
the orange, then peel and roughly chop the
ginger.

2. Transfer to a blender with the dates
and ⅔ cup (160 ml) water and blend until
creamy. Pour into a glass and enjoy.

Banana-Kiwi Smoothie

SERVES 1
PREP TIME: 10 minutes
PER SERVING: 215 calories, 4 g protein,
1 g fat, 44 g carbohydrates

1 banana
2 kiwis
1 orange
½ bunch parsley

1. Peel the banana and kiwis. Peel and slice
the orange. Roughly chop the parsley.

2. Transfer to a blender with a scant ½ cup
(100 ml) water and blend until creamy.
Pour into a glass and enjoy.

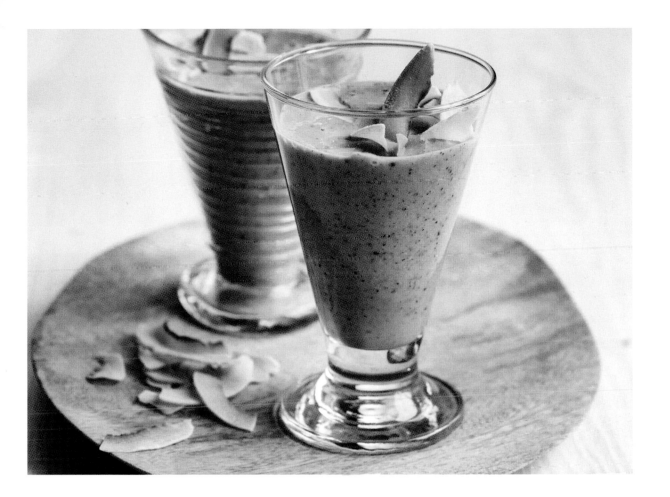

Vanilla Oat Shake

SERVES 1
PREP TIME: 15 minutes
PER SERVING: 480 calories, 15 g protein,
21 g fat, 58 g carbohydrates

⅓ cup (30 g) rolled oats
1 tablespoon chia seeds
Scant 1 cup (200 ml) boiling water
1 banana
1 tablespoon shredded coconut
1 teaspoon ground cinnamon
½ teaspoon bourbon vanilla extract
Scant 1 cup (200 ml) Almond Milk
  (page 145)

1. In a medium bowl, combine the oats and chia seeds. Add the boiling water, stir, and soak for 10 minutes.

2. Drain the oat mixture of any water that hasn't been absorbed and transfer to a blender. Peel the banana and add it to the blender with the remaining ingredients, then blend until creamy. Pour into a glass, top with additional coconut, if desired, and enjoy.

Homemade Plant Milk

It's easy to make your own plant milk, and making your own means avoiding all the added sugar, stabilizers, and emulsifiers that are often found in store-bought milk. You can even save leftover nut meal to make nut butter or Energy Balls (page 262). Simply follow these steps after soaking the nuts or oats.

- Drain and transfer to a blender with 4 cups (1 L) water and blend.

- Carefully press out the liquid through a very fine sieve or nut milk bag.

- Pour the milk into a bottle or pitcher and store in the refrigerator before serving.

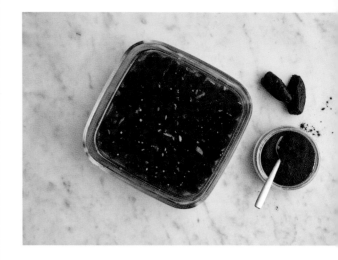

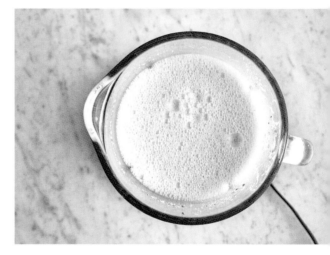

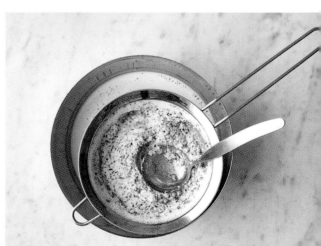

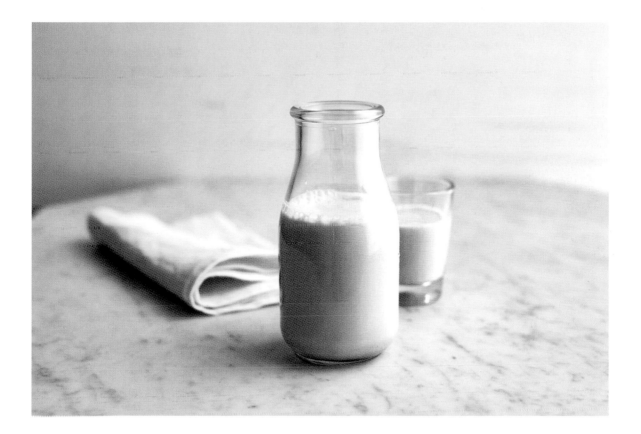

Almond Milk

MAKES 4 CUPS (1 L)
PREP TIME: 5 minutes
SOAKING TIME: 6 hours (or overnight)
PER SERVING (½ CUP/100 ML): 50 calories,
2 g protein, 4 g fat, 2 g carbohydrates

1⅓ cups (200 g) raw almonds
2 Medjool dates, pitted
1 teaspoon ground cinnamon, optional

---

1. Soak the almonds in water for at least 6 hours (or overnight).

2. Follow the steps for making plant milk, blending the almonds with the dates and cinnamon, if using, for 2 minutes.

Cashew Milk

MAKES 4 CUPS (1 L)
PREP TIME: 5 minutes
SOAKING TIME: 3 hours
PER SERVING (½ CUP/100 ML): 50 calories,
1 g protein, 3 g fat, 3 g carbohydrates

1½ cups (200 g) raw cashews
Agave syrup, optional

---

1. Soak the cashews for at least 3 hours.

2. Follow the steps for making plant milk, blending for 1 minute and sweetening with agave syrup, if desired.

Oat Milk

MAKES 4 CUPS (1 L)
PREP TIME: 5 minutes
SOAKING TIME: 30 minutes
PER SERVING (½ CUP/100 ML): 60 calories,
2 g protein, 1 g fat, 9 g carbohydrates

2¼ cups (200 g) rolled oats
Agave syrup, optional

---

1. Soak the oats for at least 30 minutes.

2. Follow the steps for making plant milk, blending for 2 minutes and sweetening with agave syrup, if desired.

Ayurvedic Golden Milk (*Haldi doodh*)

SERVES 2
PREP TIME: 10 minutes
PER SERVING: 190 calories, 3 g protein, 6 g fat,
30 g carbohydrates

---

2 cups (500 ml) Almond Milk (page 145)
1 tablespoon ground cinnamon
1 tablespoon ground turmeric
1 teaspoon ground cardamom
1 teaspoon coconut nectar or maple syrup
½ teaspoon Bourbon vanilla extract

---

1. Stir all the ingredients together in a medium pot and bring to a boil, then remove from the heat.

2. Strain the milk through a fine sieve into two mugs.

3. Froth with a milk frother, if desired. Enjoy warm or cold.

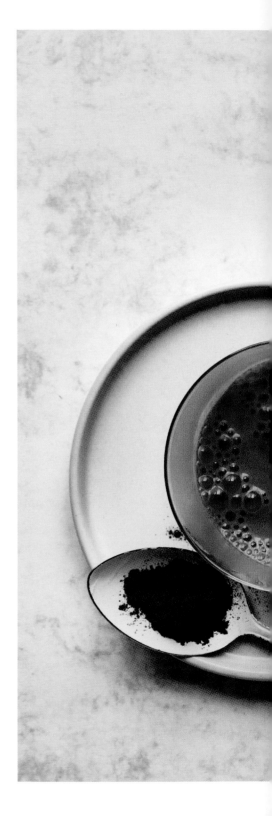

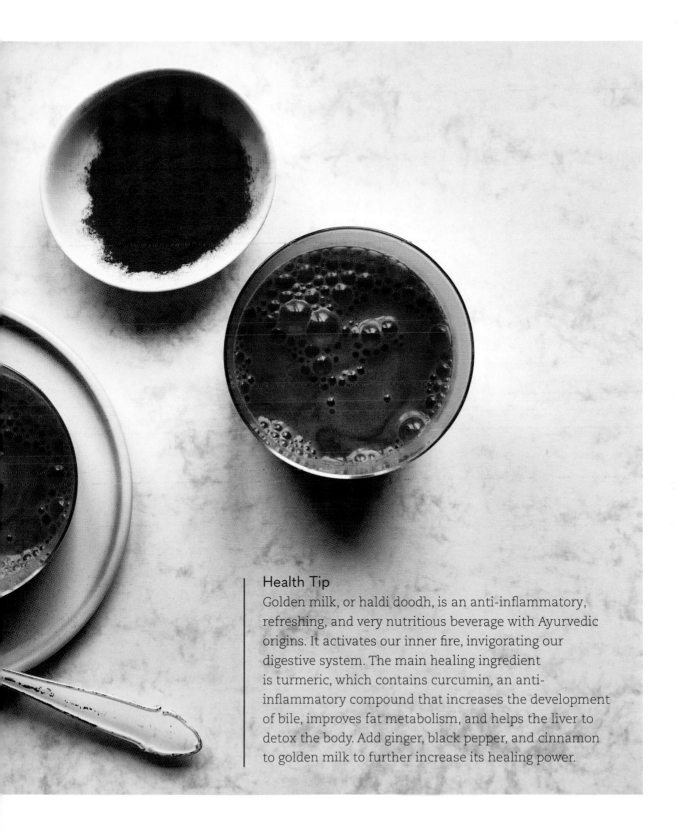

Health Tip

Golden milk, or haldi doodh, is an anti-inflammatory, refreshing, and very nutritious beverage with Ayurvedic origins. It activates our inner fire, invigorating our digestive system. The main healing ingredient is turmeric, which contains curcumin, an anti-inflammatory compound that increases the development of bile, improves fat metabolism, and helps the liver to detox the body. Add ginger, black pepper, and cinnamon to golden milk to further increase its healing power.

Berry-Coconut Chia Pudding

SERVES 1
PREP TIME: 5 minutes
SOAKING TIME: 1 hour
PER SERVING: 410 calories, 10 g protein,
26 g fat, 34 g carbohydrates

---

2 tablespoons chia seeds

2 tablespoons coconut milk

Scant ½ cup (100 g) coconut yogurt

1 teaspoon coconut nectar or maple
   syrup

½ teaspoon ground cinnamon

1 small handful fresh berries

1 tablespoon cacao nibs

---

1. In a medium bowl, combine the chia seeds with the coconut milk and ⅔ cup (160 ml) water. Let the mixture soak for at least 1 hour.

2. Add half of the yogurt, the coconut nectar, and cinnamon, and stir thoroughly.

3. Garnish with the rest of the yogurt, berries, and cacao nibs.

Health Tip
Chia seeds contain five times as much calcium as cow's milk, as well as many omega-3 fatty acids. The antioxidants protect our cells from free radicals, making chia seeds a true superfood.

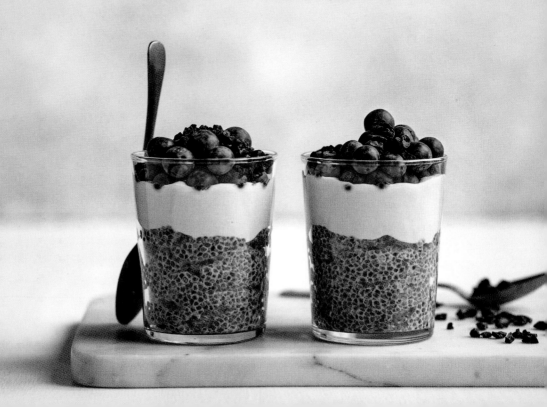

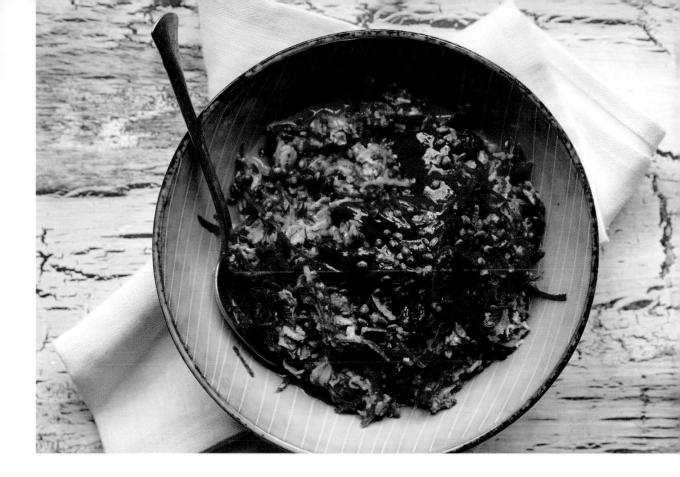

Cinnamon-Carrot Overnight Oats

SERVES 2
PREP TIME: 10 minutes
SOAKING TIME: 1 hour
PER SERVING: 370 calories, 11 g protein,
20 g fat, 39 g carbohydrates

⅓ cup (30 g) rolled oats
¾ cup (180 ml) Almond Milk (page 145)
1 apple
1 carrot
1 tablespoon raisins
1 teaspoon ground cinnamon
½ teaspoon ground cardamom
2 tablespoons Almond Butter (page 150)
1 tablespoon hemp seeds

---

1. Mix the oats with the milk and let them soak in the refrigerator for at least 1 hour.

2. Quarter, core, and grate the apple, then finely grate the carrot. Add to the oat mixture along with the raisins, cinnamon, and cardamom. Stir to combine.

3. Divide between two small bowls, top with the almond butter and hemp seeds, and serve.

Health Tip
The essential oils in cardamom have a positive effect on the stomach and intestines, furthering digestion and banishing bloating.

Almond Butter

MAKES ABOUT 2 CUPS (455 G)
PREP TIME: 45 minutes
PER SERVING (1 TABLESPOON): 85 calories, 3 g protein, 8 g fat, 1 g carbohydrates

---

1 pound (455 g) almonds
  (about 3 cups)

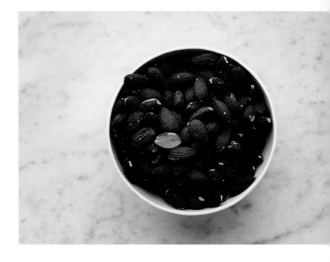

1. Preheat the oven to 350°F (180°C).

2. Roast the almonds on a dry baking sheet for 8 to 10 minutes, until fragrant. Remove from the oven and let cool.

3. Transfer to a food processor or blender and blend until creamy, pausing to scrape down the sides if necessary.

4. Store in a jar or airtight container. It will keep for about 3 weeks in the refrigerator.

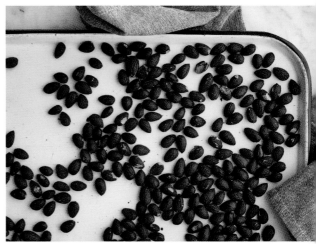

NOTE: If you like your almond butter a bit sweeter, fold in 1 tablespoon coconut sugar, 2 teaspoons ground cinnamon, and a pinch of sea salt after blending.

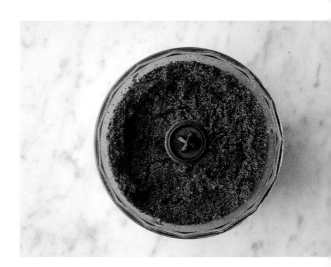

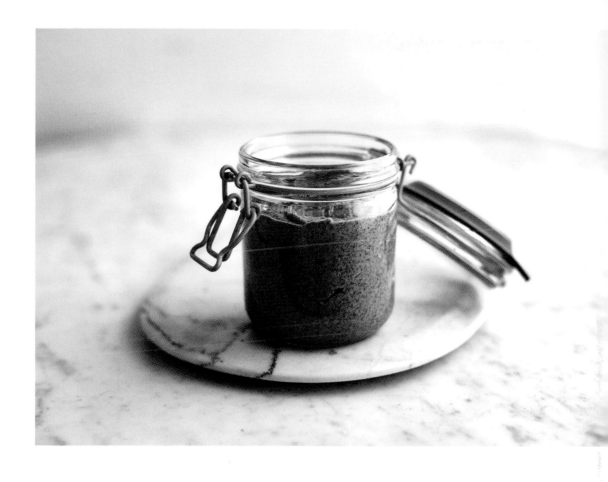

Health Tip

Almonds contain lots of simple unsaturated fatty acids and large amounts of potassium, magnesium, and calcium—more so than other nuts. They are also an excellent source of B vitamins, folic acid, secondary phytochemicals, and fiber.

Almond butter is also said to have prebiotic properties—it supports the growth of the healthy bacteria in the intestine. It's also excellent for regulating blood sugar and cholesterol levels.

Almond butter is a healthy alternative to store-bought chocolate hazelnut spreads (think: Nutella) and, of course, to butter made from cow's milk. You can also use it to thicken sauces and curries or to give salad dressings a nutty flavor.

Zucchini Porridge

SERVES 2
PREP TIME: 15 minutes
PER SERVING: 180 calories, 6 g protein,
2 g fat, 33 g carbohydrates

---

1 zucchini
½ cup (45 g) rolled oats
1 teaspoon ground cinnamon
1 banana
1 tablespoon maple syrup

---

1. Finely grate the zucchini into a medium pot and add the oats, cinnamon, and ⅔ cup (160 ml) water. Bring to a boil, turn the heat to low, and simmer for 5 minutes, or until the water has evaporated.

2. Peel and slice the banana.

3. Divide between two bowls. Top with the banana and drizzle with the maple syrup.

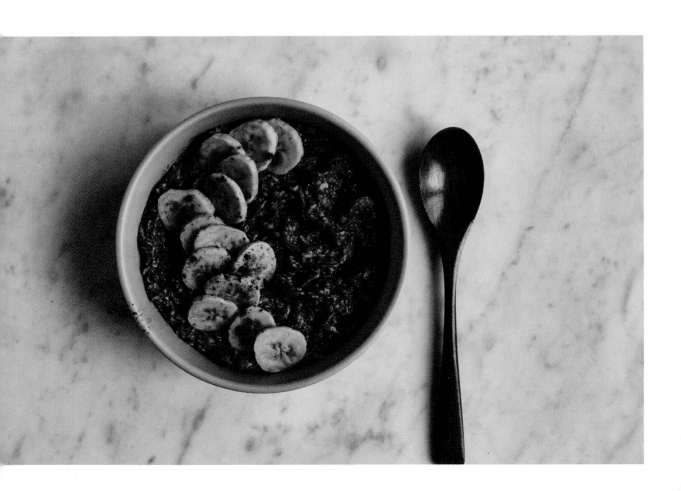

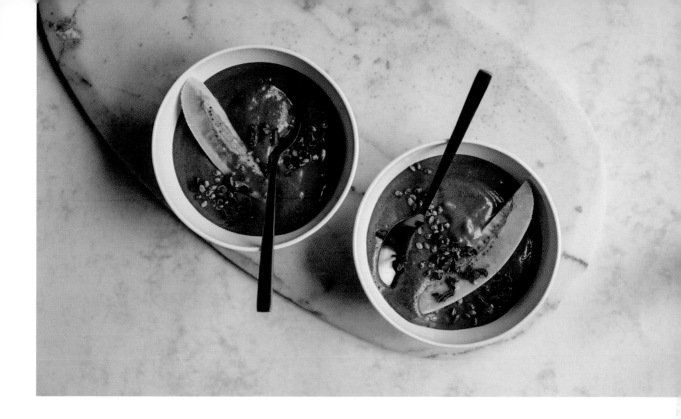

Chocolate-Banana Bowl

SERVES 2
PREP TIME: 10 minutes, plus overnight soaking
PER SERVING: 540 calories, 16 g protein,
37 g fat, 36 g carbohydrates

1½ small bananas
⅓ cup (50 g) raw cashews, soaked overnight
3 tablespoons raw almonds, soaked overnight
2 Medjool dates, pitted
2 tablespoons Almond Butter (page 150)
2 tablespoons raw cacao powder
⅓ cup (80 ml) Oat Milk (page 146)
1 tablespoon hemp seeds
2 tablespoons cacao nibs

1. Peel the bananas, then cut half a banana into slices and set aside. Blend the other banana in a blender with the cashews, almonds, dates, almond butter, cacao powder, and milk until creamy.

2. Divide between two bowls. Garnish with the banana slices, hemp seeds, and cacao nibs and serve.

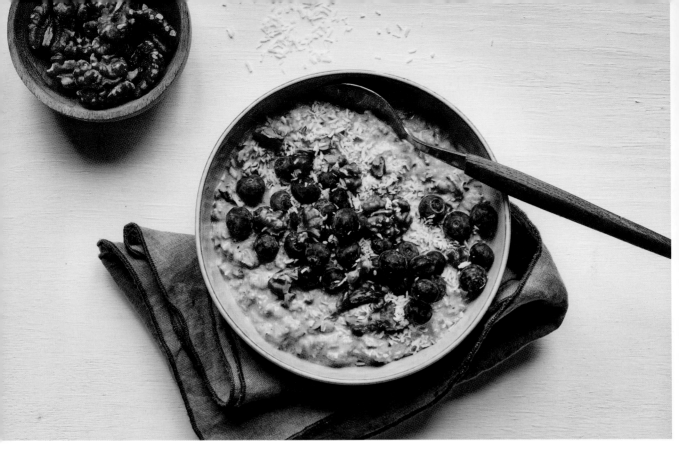

Coconut Overnight Oats

SERVES 2
PREP TIME: 10 minutes
SOAKING TIME: 1 hour
PER SERVING: 310 calories, 11 g protein,
15 g fat, 32 g carbohydrates

⅓ cup (30 g) rolled oats
¾ cup (180 ml) coconut milk
1 apple
¾ cup (200 g) unsweetened soy yogurt
1 teaspoon ground cinnamon
2 tablespoons fresh blueberries
6 walnuts
1 tablespoon shredded coconut

1. Combine the oats with the coconut milk in a small bowl and let soak in the refrigerator for at least 1 hour.

2. Quarter, core, and finely grate the apple into the soaked oats and stir to combine. Stir in the yogurt and cinnamon.

3. Divide between two bowls. Top with the blueberries, walnuts, and coconut and serve.

Health Tip
The basic ingredients in soy yogurt are soybeans and water. When purchasing soy yogurt, make sure that it doesn't contain any unnecessary artificial additives, stabilizers, flavorings, thickening agents, and, above all, sugar.

Strawberry-Basil Bowl

SERVES 2
PREP TIME: 10 minutes
PER SERVING: 230 calories, 8 g protein,
11 g fat, 24 g carbohydrates

---

2 large handfuls strawberries
1 banana
½ bunch basil
2 tablespoons flaxseeds
2 tablespoons rolled oats
¾ cup (180 ml) Almond Milk (page 145)
1 tablespoon cacao nibs

---

1. Blend the strawberries (reserving 3 berries), banana, basil (reserving a few leaves), flaxseeds, oats, and milk in a blender until creamy.

2. Divide between two bowls. Cut the reserved strawberries into slices, lay them on the bowls, and top with the cacao nibs and reserved basil leaves.

NOTE: If you don't like bananas, you can use an avocado, which makes this bowl even creamier.

Health Tip
Although strawberries are 90 percent water, they still pack a real punch. They have twice as much vitamin C as oranges, few carbohydrates, and nearly no fat. They also have a strong antioxidant effect: They protect the cells from free radicals and help to reduce high blood pressure.

The basil may seem to be an unusual choice here, but its bright flavor accentuates the sweetness of the strawberries. The bright green leaves contain many vital ingredients, particularly beta carotene, the precursor to vitamin A, as well as calcium, iron, and vitamin K. The essential oils found in basil have an anti-inflammatory effect and are antibacterial.

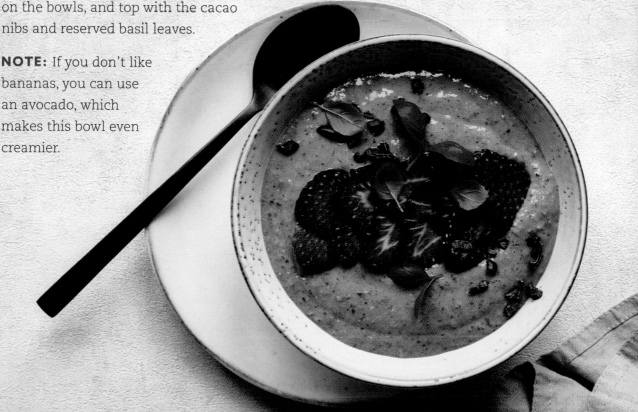

Breakfast Muffins

MAKES 6 MUFFINS, SERVES 1 EACH
PREP TIME: 25 minutes
BAKING TIME: 30 minutes
PER SERVING: 210 calories, 5 g protein, 13 g fat,
18 g carbohydrates

1⅓ cups (120 g) rolled oats
2 tablespoons pumpkin seeds
1 tablespoon ground poppy seeds
1 tablespoon ground cinnamon
1 teaspoon baking powder
1 very ripe banana
½ cup plus 1 tablespoon (130 ml) Almond
    Milk (page 145)
2½ tablespoons (40 g) canola oil, plus extra
    for greasing

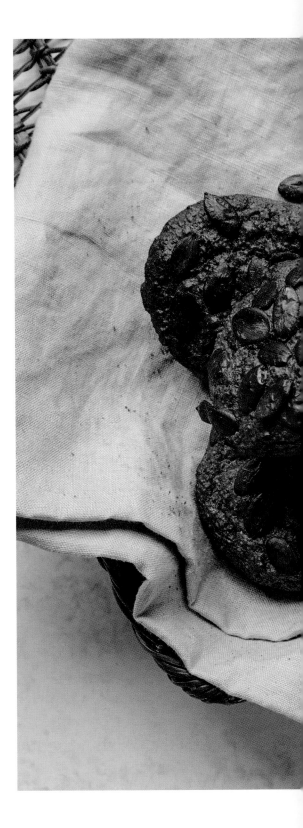

1. Preheat the oven to 400 °F (200°C). Grease
six cups of a muffin pan.

2. Finely grind the oats in a food processor.

3. Transfer to a medium bowl and mix in the
pumpkin seeds, poppy seeds, cinnamon, and
baking powder.

4. Peel and mash the banana with a fork.
Transfer to a large bowl and add the milk and
oil. Mix well.

5. Add the dry ingredients gradually to the wet
ingredients. Mix until a smooth batter forms.

6. Spoon into the muffin pan cups. Bake
on the middle rack for 30 minutes, or until
golden brown.

7. Remove from the oven and let cool in the
pan for 5 minutes, then carefully remove the
muffins and let cool on a wire rack before
serving.

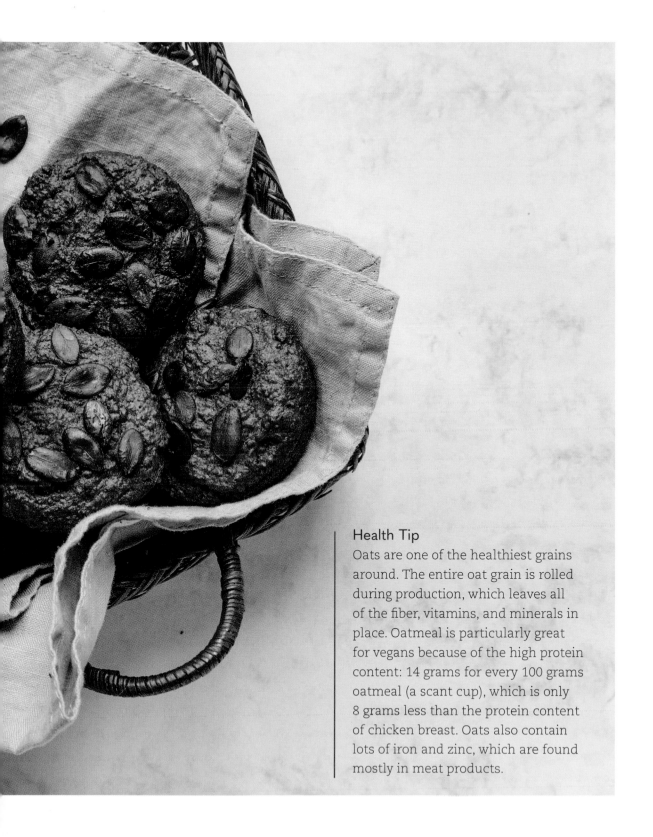

Health Tip

Oats are one of the healthiest grains around. The entire oat grain is rolled during production, which leaves all of the fiber, vitamins, and minerals in place. Oatmeal is particularly great for vegans because of the high protein content: 14 grams for every 100 grams oatmeal (a scant cup), which is only 8 grams less than the protein content of chicken breast. Oats also contain lots of iron and zinc, which are found mostly in meat products.

Pumpkin Seed and Chia Bread

MAKES ONE 9 × 5-INCH (23 × 13 CM) LOAF
PREP TIME: 15 minutes, plus 2 hours resting time
BAKING TIME: 60 minutes
PER SERVING (½-INCH/1 CM SLICE):
300 calories, 14 g protein, 11 g fat, 34 g
carbohydrates

---

1 tablespoon coconut sugar
2½ teaspoons (one ¼-ounce/7 g packet)
    active dry yeast
2 cups (500 ml) warm water
3⅔ cups (440 g) spelt flour
½ cup (60 g) pumpkin seeds
½ cup (60 g) pumpkin seed powder
⅓ cup (50 g) flaxseeds
⅓ cup (50 g) sesame seeds
¼ cup (30 g) sunflower seeds
2 tablespoons (20 g) chia seeds
2 teaspoons sea salt
Oil, for greasing

---

1. Combine the sugar and yeast in a small
bowl. Add the water, stir, and set aside for
5 to 10 minutes, until the mixture becomes
frothy.

2. Combine the remaining ingredients in a
medium bowl.

3. Add the yeast mixture and use a
handheld mixer to blend into a smooth,
slightly sticky dough. Cover the bowl with
a kitchen towel and let the dough rest at
room temperature for 2 hours.

4. Preheat the oven to 400°F (200°C). Grease
a 9 x 5-inch (23 x 13 cm) loaf pan with oil.

5. Transfer the dough to the pan and
smooth the top. Bake for 50 minutes.

6. Remove from the oven and carefully
remove the bread from the pan. Place the
bread back in the oven and let it bake
"naked" for another 10 minutes, or until
golden brown. Allow the bread to cool
before eating.

Health Tip

Pumpkin seed powder or flour, which
has a nutty taste, is a by-product of
the production of pumpkin seed oil.
Like pumpkin seeds themselves, this
flour has loads of potassium and
magnesium, both of which are good for
the muscles and the nervous system.
With its high fiber content, it helps to
slow down the digestive process and
keep the blood sugar low.

This bread will leave you satisfied for
a long time. But because pumpkin seed
powder doesn't contain any gluten, we
do need a certain amount of "normal"
flour (in this case, spelt) to keep the
bread from falling apart. Try pumpkin
seed powder in recipes instead of bread
crumbs and as a protein powder in
smoothies and shakes.

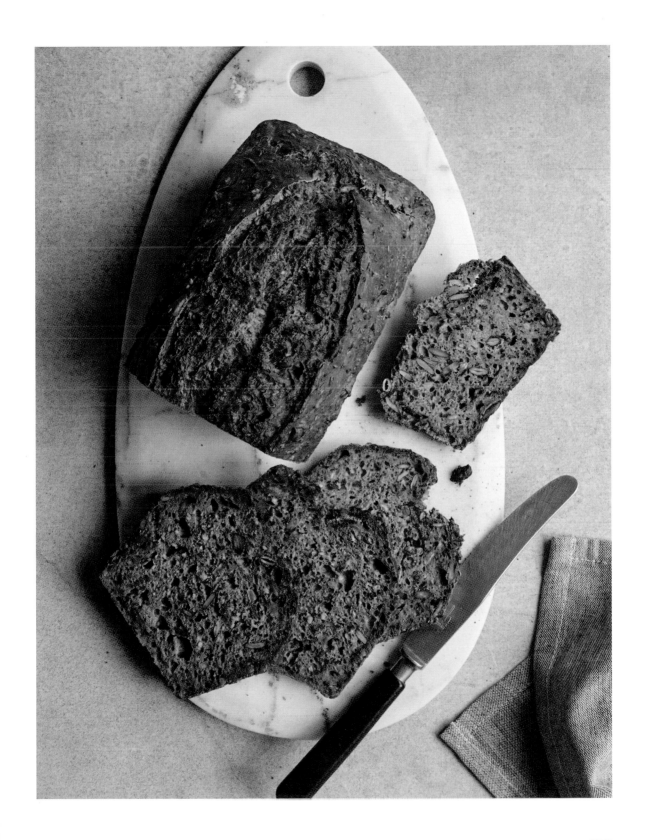

Lunch

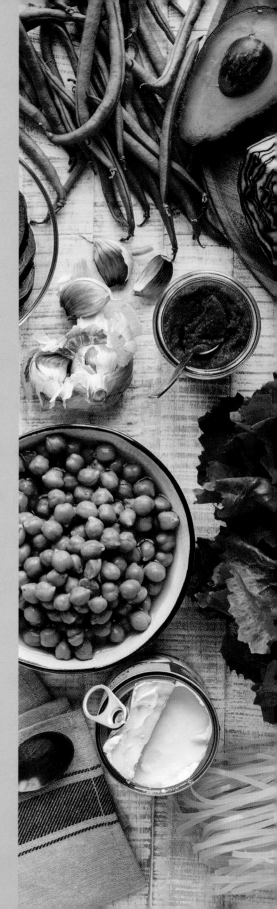

Baba Ghanoush Salad

Endive-Pear Salad

Brussels Sprout, Radicchio, and Apple Salad

Greek Salad with Rice and Lentils

Potato, Beet, and Spinach Salad

Escarole and Wild Rice Bowl

Kale-Coconut Millet Bowl

Vegetable Broth Paste

Rice Noodle Salad

Herby Buckwheat Tabbouleh

Rainbow Summer Rolls with Almond Chili Dip

Classic Hummus

Green Pea Hummus

Beet Hummus

Tomato-Lentil Tapenade

Basil Pesto

Vegetable Pasta with Avocado Sauce

Garlic-Zucchini Spaghetti

Butternut Squash Bake

Baked Sweet Potato with Guacamole

Red Squash and Fennel Stew

Potato-Mushroom Stew

Coconut-Kale Risotto

Mediterranean Tomato-Bean Sauté

Rainbow Roasted Root Vegetables

Shakshuka with Avocado

Potato-Leek Soup

Thai Coconut Noodle Soup

Baba Ghanoush Salad

SERVES 2
PREP TIME: 50 minutes
PER SERVING: 385 calories, 10 g protein, 12 g fat, 57 g carbohydrates

2 eggplants
1 tablespoon olive oil
⅓ cup (75 g) brown rice
1 red bell pepper
1 red onion
½ bunch parsley
3 tablespoons walnuts
1 tablespoon ground cumin
¼ cup (40 g) pomegranate seeds, optional

DRESSING

¼ cup (60 ml) lemon juice
2 tablespoons agave syrup
Sea salt
Fresh ground black pepper
Chili paste, optional

1. Preheat the oven to 450°F (240°C).

2. Halve the eggplants lengthwise, then use a fork to prick the skin all over. Brush them with the oil, then place them on a baking sheet, cut side down, and bake for 30 minutes (turning once after 15 minutes).

3. Meanwhile, cook the rice according to the package instructions. Finely dice the bell pepper. Peel and finely dice the onion. Finely chop the parsley and walnuts.

4. Remove the eggplants from the oven and let cool, then peel off the skin.

5. Transfer to a medium bowl and mash with a fork. Add the onion and bell pepper. Stir to combine, then mix in the parsley, walnuts, and cumin.

6. To make the dressing, mix the lemon juice and agave syrup in a small bowl. Season with salt, pepper, and chili paste, if using.

7. Pour the dressing over the baba ghanoush. Serve with the rice and garnish with pomegranate seeds, if using.

Health Tip

Eggplants contain almost no calories but lots of B vitamins, vitamin C, and potassium—an amazing combination for your heart and cardiovascular system. They're also rich in antioxidants and have a diuretic effect.

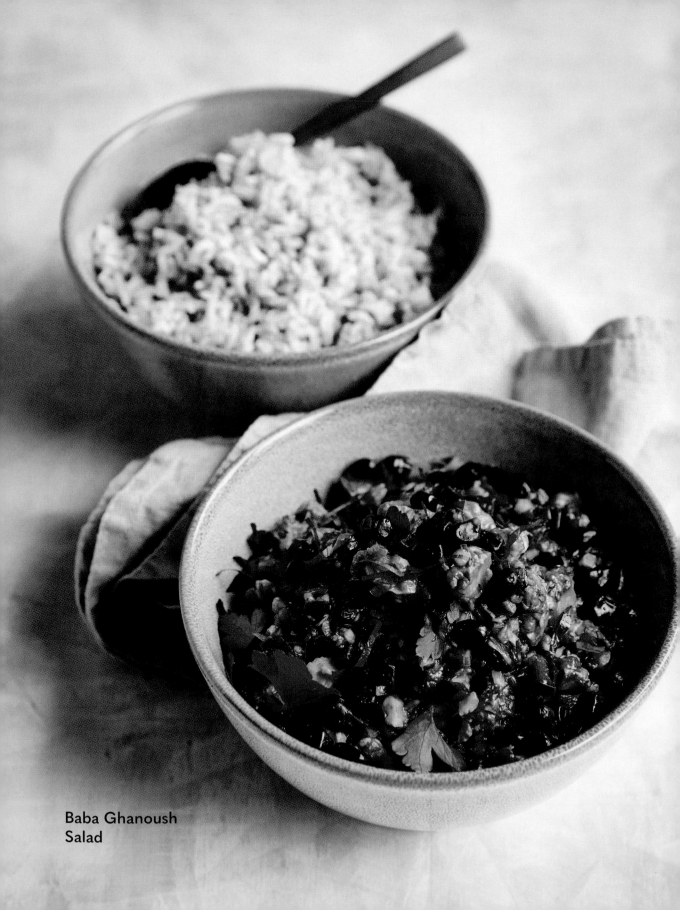

Baba Ghanoush
Salad

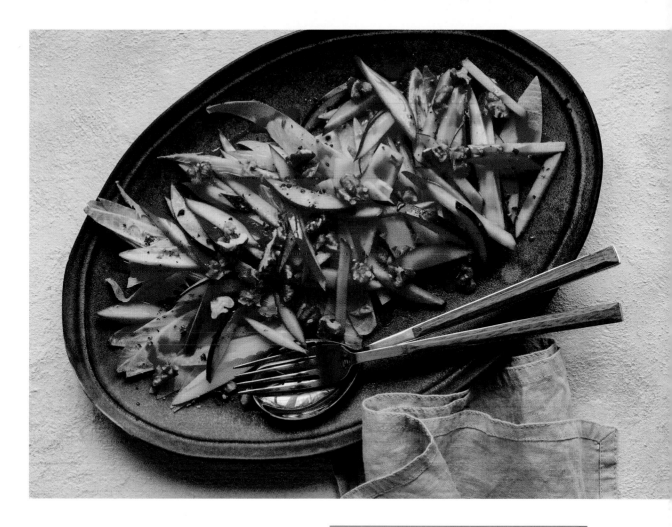

Endive-Pear Salad

SERVES 2
PREP TIME: 20 minutes
PER SERVING: 400 calories, 7 g protein,
27 g fat, 31 g carbohydrates

11 ounces (300 g) Belgian endive (about
3 to 4)

2 juicy pears

1 apple

½ cup (50 g) walnuts

DRESSING

2 tablespoons walnut oil

2 tablespoons white wine vinegar

1 teaspoon agave syrup

1 teaspoon Dijon mustard

Sea salt

Fresh ground black pepper

(recipe continues . . .)

1. Cut off and discard the endive stems. Cut the leaves into bite-size slivers.

2. Core the pears and apple and cut them into thin sticks. Coarsely chop the walnuts.

3. Combine the endive, pears, apple, and walnuts in a medium bowl.

4. To make the dressing, combine the oil, vinegar, agave syrup, and mustard in a small bowl and stir until creamy. Season with salt and pepper.

5. Toss the salad with the dressing, then divide between bowls and enjoy.

> ### Health Tip
> Endive has an intense, bitter flavor to it, and it's very healthy: The bitter substances stimulate fat burning, support the liver in detoxification, enhance digestion, and strengthen the immune system. The high levels of beta carotene and potassium help ramp up cell regeneration. The vitamin C also strengthens blood vessels. And because endive contains inulin, a prebiotic fiber, it also promotes the growth of "good" intestinal bacteria and keeps us feeling full for a long time.

Brussels Sprout, Radicchio, and Apple Salad

SERVES 2
PREP TIME: 20 minutes
PER SERVING: 450 calories, 11 g protein, 35 g fat, 22 g carbohydrates

---

7 ounces (200 g) brussels sprouts (about 2¼ cups)
½ head radicchio
2 apples
⅓ cup (45 g) almonds

DRESSING
¼ cup (60 ml) olive oil
2 tablespoons apple cider vinegar
2 teaspoons mustard
Sea salt
Fresh ground black pepper

---

1. Remove the outer leaves of the brussels sprouts and cut off the hard ends, then thinly slice them. Transfer to a medium bowl.

2. Tear the radicchio into bite-size pieces. Quarter, core, and finely dice the apple. Add to the bowl with the sprouts.

3. Toast the almonds in a dry skillet over medium until they are fragrant, about 5 minutes.

4. To make the dressing, mix the oil, vinegar, and mustard in a small bowl. Season with salt and pepper.

5. Toss the salad with the dressing and top with the almonds. Divide between bowls and serve.

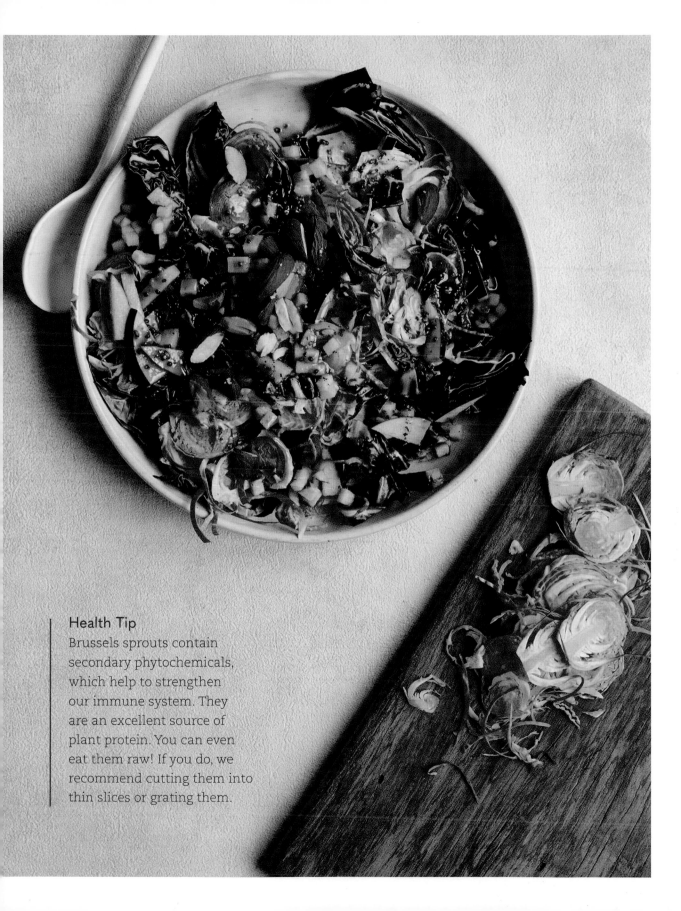

Health Tip

Brussels sprouts contain
secondary phytochemicals,
which help to strengthen
our immune system. They
are an excellent source of
plant protein. You can even
eat them raw! If you do, we
recommend cutting them into
thin slices or grating them.

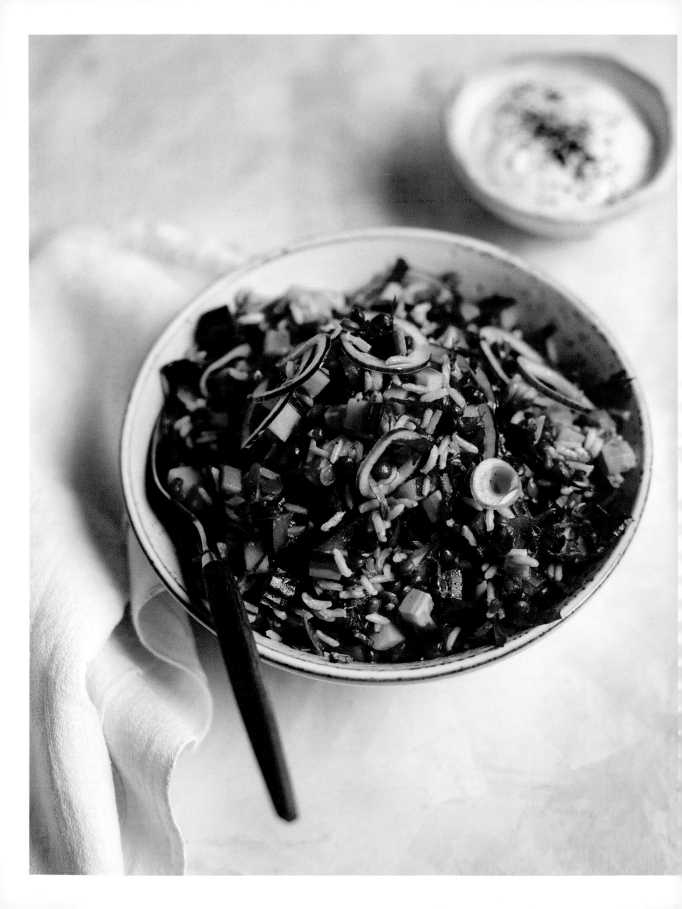

Greek Salad with Rice and Lentils

SERVES 2
PREP TIME: 30 minutes
PER SERVING: 810 calories, 27 g protein, 29 g fat, 102 g carbohydrates

¾ cup (150 g) brown basmati rice
¾ cup (150 g) brown lentils
1 small red onion
1 large tomato
1 cucumber
½ bunch cilantro
½ bunch mint
2 tablespoons unsweetened soy yogurt
Red pepper flakes, optional

DRESSING
⅓ cup (80 ml) olive oil
Juice of 1 lemon
Sea salt
Fresh ground black pepper

1. Rinse the rice, then cook according to the package instructions. Rinse the lentils, then cook according to the package instructions. Set aside to cool.

2. Meanwhile, peel the onion and slice into fine rings. Finely dice the tomato and cucumber. Finely chop the cilantro and mint.

3. To make the dressing, mix the oil and lemon juice in a small bowl and season with salt and pepper.

4. Combine the rice, lentils, onion, tomato, cucumber, and herbs in a medium bowl. Pour in the dressing and stir to combine. Garnish with the yogurt and red pepper flakes, if using, and serve.

Potato, Beet, and Spinach Salad

SERVES 2
PREP TIME: 30 minutes
PER SERVING: 530 calories, 11 g protein, 34 g fat, 41 g carbohydrates

Sea salt
4 small waxy potatoes
2 fresh medium beets (about 7 ounces/200 g)
7 ounces (200 g) baby spinach
2 tablespoons dried cranberries
1 handful walnuts

DRESSING
3 tablespoons apple cider vinegar
3 tablespoons walnut oil
Juice of ½ lemon
1 teaspoon agave syrup
Sea salt
Fresh ground black pepper

1. Bring a medium pot of salted water to a boil. Peel and dice the potatoes, then add to the pot and cook for 10 to 15 minutes, until fork tender. Peel and dice the beets.

2. Drain and transfer the potatoes to a medium bowl. Add the beets and spinach.

3. To make the dressing, mix the vinegar, oil, lemon juice, and agave syrup in a small bowl. Season with salt and pepper.

4. Pour the dressing over the salad and toss. Top with the cranberries and walnuts, then divide between bowls and serve.

Health Tip
Beets are an amazing vegetable: They protect the heart and the blood vessels and can even help lower high blood pressure. They contain many secondary phytochemicals that can strengthen the liver and the gallbladder. You can relieve many digestion problems by regularly eating a serving of red beets. And because they contain folic acid, they are especially great for pregnant women.

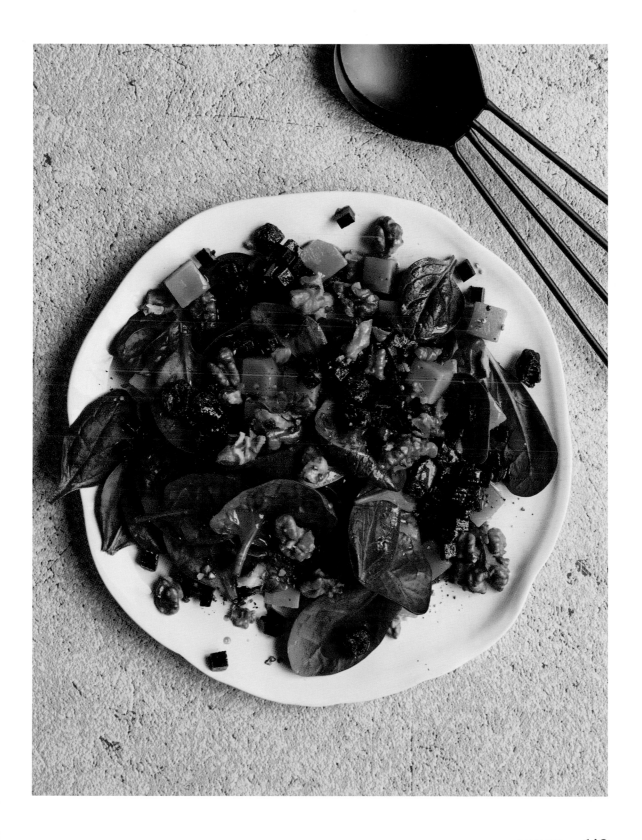

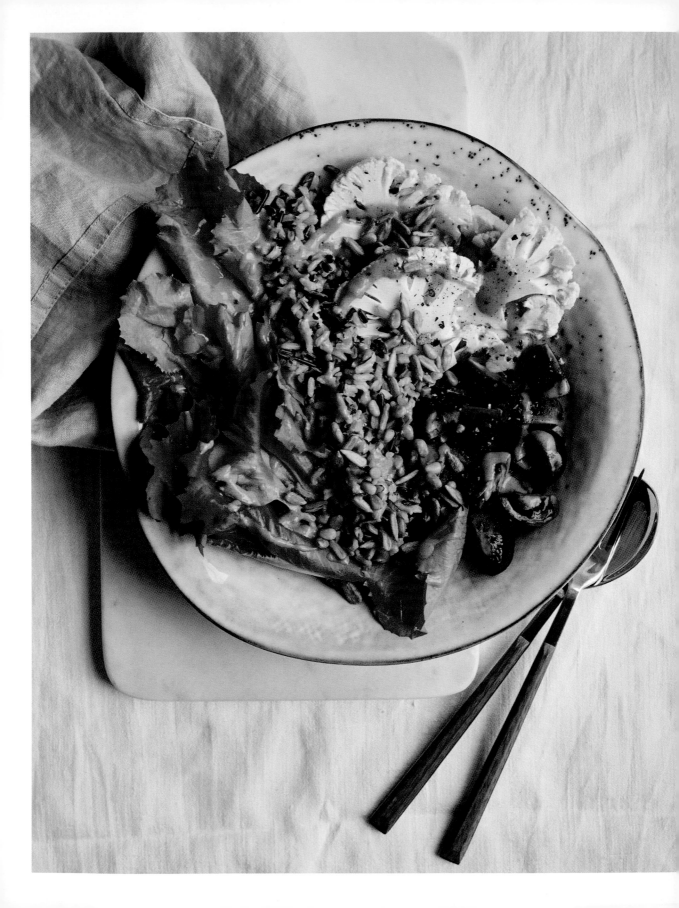

Escarole and Wild Rice Bowl

SERVES 2
PREP TIME: 50 minutes
PER SERVING: 660 calories, 18 g protein, 28 g fat, 84 g carbohydrates

1¼ cups (200 g) wild rice
½ head escarole
½ head cauliflower
10 cherry tomatoes
2 tablespoons mixed seeds (such as sesame, pumpkin, sunflower, or chia)

DRESSING
3 tablespoons olive oil
Juice of ½ lemon
1 tablespoon tahini
1 teaspoon ground cumin
Sea salt
Fresh ground black pepper

1. Cook the wild rice according to the package instructions.

2. Meanwhile, tear the escarole leaves into bite-size pieces, break the cauliflower into florets, and quarter the cherry tomatoes.

3. Divide the vegetables between two bowls. Fill one quarter of each bowl with the cauliflower, one with the escarole, one with the tomatoes, and finish with the wild rice.

4. To make the dressing, mix the oil, lemon juice, tahini, and cumin in a small bowl until creamy. Season with salt and pepper.

5. Sprinkle the dressing on the bowls and garnish with the seeds.

Health Tip
Strictly speaking, wild rice is not rice at all but the seed of a North American water grass. Like brown rice, it's considerably healthier than white rice. It contains, for example, a ton of protein (14 grams per 100 grams rice) and is rich in essential amino acids. It also has twice the amount of riboflavin (vitamin B_2) and niacin (vitamin B_3) as white rice.

Kale-Coconut Millet Bowl

SERVES 2
PREP TIME: 40 minutes
PER SERVING: 745 calories, 19 g protein, 53 g fat, 46 g carbohydrates

---

1 zucchini
5 large kale leaves
1 bunch parsley
½ cup (100 g) millet
¾ cup (180 ml) coconut milk
2 tablespoons Almond Butter (page 150)
2 tablespoons olive oil
2 tablespoons tahini
Juice of ½ lemon
1 teaspoon Vegetable Broth Paste
   (page 174)
1 teaspoon ground cumin
Fresh ground black pepper

---

1. Dice the zucchini, then stem and thinly slice the kale. Finely chop the parsley.

2. Rinse the millet thoroughly under running cold water and cook according to the package instructions.

3. Transfer the kale and zucchini to a medium pot. Add the coconut milk and bring the mixture to a boil. Add the almond butter, oil, tahini, lemon juice, broth paste, and cumin, reduce the heat, and simmer for 2 minutes. Season with salt and pepper.

4. Divide the millet and vegetables between two bowls and serve.

Health Tip

The high amount of vital ingredients in kale makes it a true superfood. For example, 100 grams of kale contain as much bone-strengthening calcium as a large glass of cow's milk, and the amount of vitamin C in kale is greater than that of all citrus fruits. It's second only to carrots as a source of provitamin A. It also contains more iron than beef, making it an ideal vegetable for both vegans and vegetarians. And it's rich in alpha-linolenic acid, an omega-3 fatty acid. Regular consumption of kale has an anti-inflammatory effect and improves blood flow, helping to prevent heart disease.

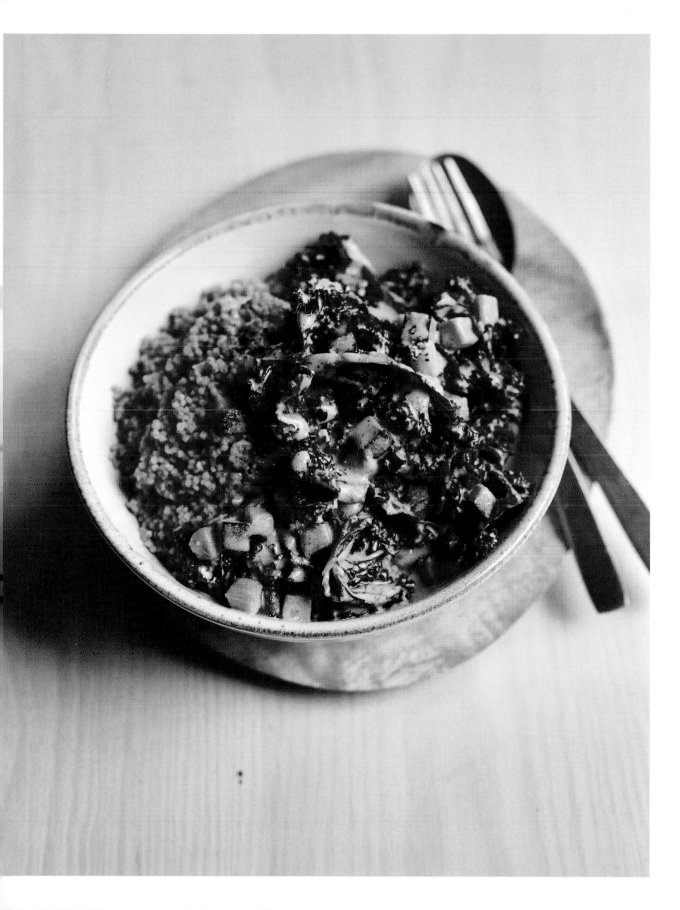

Vegetable Broth Paste

MAKES ABOUT 1½ CUPS (500 G)
PREP TIME: 15 minutes
PER SERVING (1 TABLESPOON): 3 calories,
0 g protein, 0 g fat, 0.5 g carbohydrates

---

1 cup (100 g) chopped leek
¾ cup (100 g) chopped carrots
¾ cup (100 g) chopped parsnips
⅔ cup (100 g) chopped celery root
1 cup (60 g) parsley
¼ cup plus 1 tablespoon (90 g) sea salt

---

1. Place all of the vegetables in a blender along with the parsley and salt and blend at a high speed until it becomes a smooth paste.

2. Transfer to a clean jar and store in the refrigerator. It will keep for weeks or even months—if you can keep yourself from gobbling it up!

NOTE: This paste can serve as a basis for soups, stews, curries, and much more. Just heat 4 cups (1 L) water and add 2 to 3 tablespoons paste.

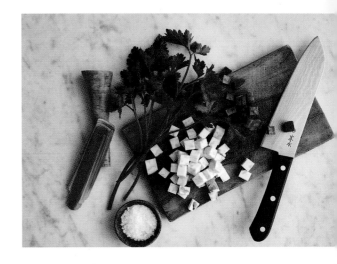

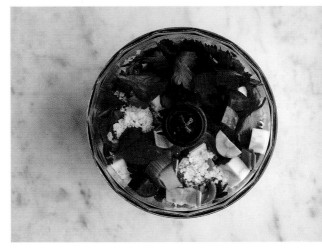

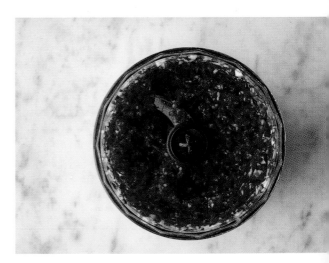

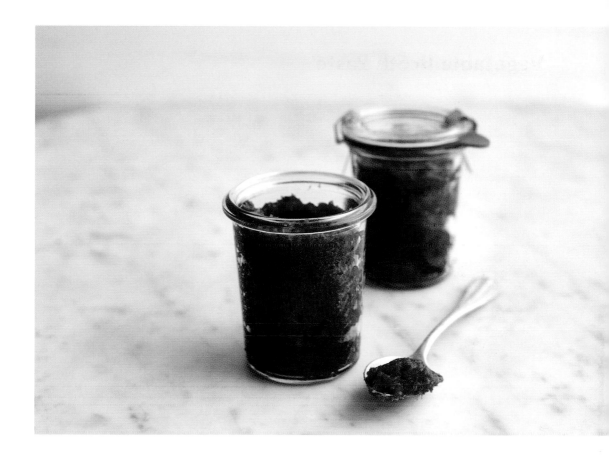

Health Tip

This homemade seasoning paste is so much healthier than the store-bought varieties, which often contain added sugar, yeast, fillers, and additives our body doesn't need. The vegetables in this recipe contain everything you need for a tasty, aromatic vegetable broth. Feel free to use whatever your refrigerator or the farmers market has to offer. Stay away from vegetables containing a lot of water, such as tomatoes and cucumbers, since their moisture will shorten the shelf life of the paste. If you like, add in herbs for more flavor: parsley, chives, dill, celery greens, carrot greens, oregano, mint, lemon balm—experiment and see what you like best.

Rice Noodle Salad

SERVES 2
PREP TIME: 30 minutes
PER SERVING: 775 calories, 22 g protein, 38 g fat, 83 g carbohydrates

---

5 ounces (150 g) wide rice noodles or glass noodles
10 ounces (300 g) chard (about 6 leaves)
2 scallions
1 carrot
¼ bunch cilantro
Red pepper flakes, optional
⅓ cup (50 g) roasted peanuts

DRESSING

1 garlic clove
Juice of 1 lime
3 tablespoons toasted sesame oil
3 tablespoons soy sauce
2 tablespoons maple syrup
2 tablespoons peanut butter

---

1. Cook the noodles according to the package instructions. Drain and rinse with cold water.

2. Thinly slice the chard, scallions, and carrot. Finely chop the cilantro.

3. To prepare the dressing, peel and finely chop the garlic and transfer to a small bowl along with the lime juice, oil, soy sauce, maple syrup, and peanut butter. Stir to combine.

4. Combine the noodles, chard, scallions, and carrot in a large bowl, then add the dressing and mix well. Season with red pepper flakes, if using. Top with the peanuts and cilantro and serve.

Health Tip

Chard has been cultivated for over four thousand years and is an excellent alternative to spinach. It contains many healthy nutrients, including beta carotene, which the body then converts to vitamin A. It's also rich in B vitamins, potassium, calcium, iron, and vitamin C.

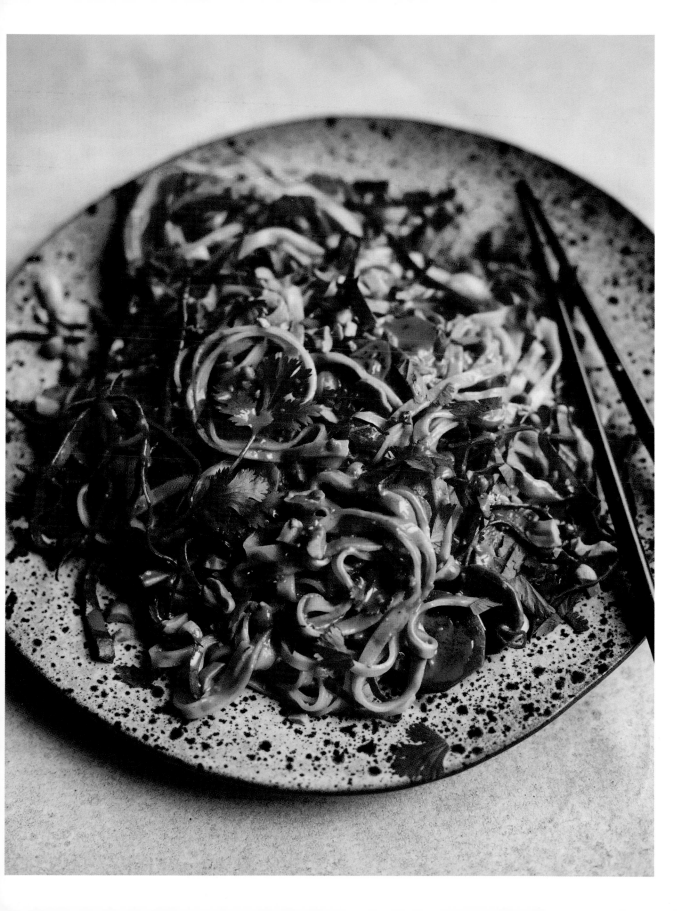

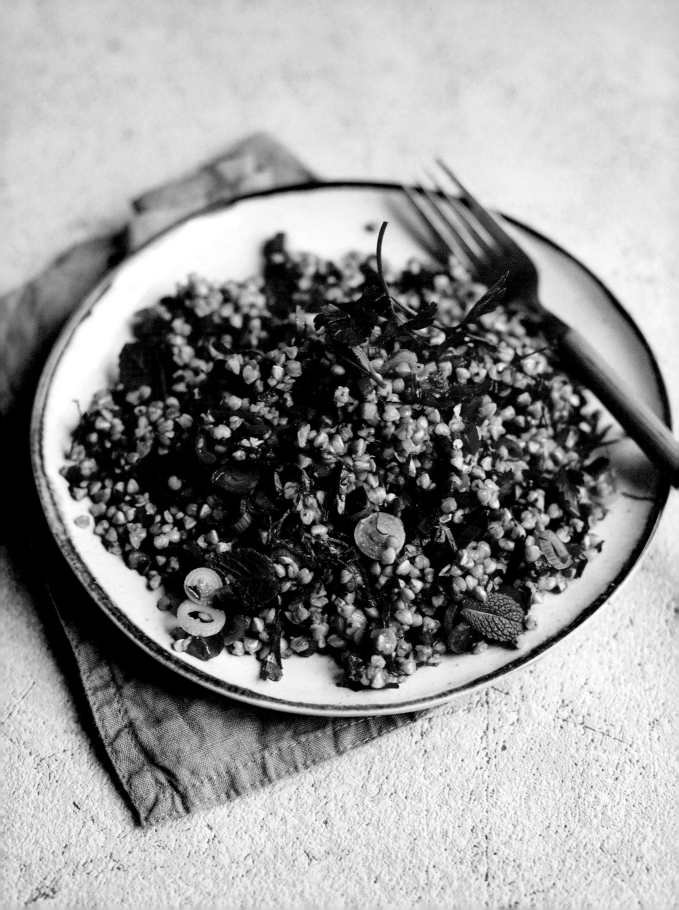

Herby Buckwheat Tabbouleh

SERVES 2
PREP TIME: 45 minutes
PER SERVING: 635 calories, 10 g protein, 28 g fat, 82 g carbohydrates

---

7 ounces (200 g) buckwheat groats
1 bunch parsley
½ bunch mint
2 scallions
2 tomatoes
1 teaspoon ground cumin
1 teaspoon paprika

DRESSING

⅓ cup (75 ml) olive oil
Juice of 1 lemon
Sea salt
Fresh ground black pepper

---

1. Cook the buckwheat according to the package instructions.

2. Finely chop the parsley and mint. Thinly slice the scallions and dice the tomatoes.

3. To prepare the dressing, mix the oil and lemon juice in a small bowl and season with salt and pepper.

4. Transfer the buckwheat, herbs, scallions, and tomatoes to a bowl, season with the cumin and paprika, and mix.

5. Pour the dressing over the salad, mix carefully, and let rest for at least 15 minutes. The longer it can rest, the better the flavors will be.

Health Tip
Like all pseudocereals, buckwheat contains no gluten and is thus a healthy alternative to wheat and other grain products. The seed can be ground to make a flour, which, like the entire grain, is rich in B vitamins.

Rainbow Summer Rolls with Almond Chili Dip

MAKES 8 ROLLS
PREP TIME: 30 minutes
PER SERVING: 130 calories, 4 g protein, 4 g fat, 19 g carbohydrates

---

3½ ounces (100 g) thin rice noodles
½ cucumber
1 small carrot
1 cup (60 g) shredded red cabbage
½ bunch mint
½ bunch cilantro
8 rice paper wrappers

DIP
3 Medjool dates, pitted
⅓ cup (80 ml) boiling water
3 tablespoons Almond Butter (page 150)
2 tablespoons soy sauce
Juice of 1 lime
1 teaspoon chili paste

---

1. Cook the noodles according to the package instructions. Drain and rinse with cold water. Set aside.

2. Julienne the cucumber and carrot.

3. To make the dip, soak the dates in the boiling water for 10 minutes. Transfer the dates and water to a blender along with the almond butter, soy sauce, lime juice, and chili paste. Blend until smooth.

4. Fill a large bowl with cold water. Soak one rice paper wrapper in the water until it becomes elastic. Transfer to a large plate.

5. Place one eighth of the vegetables, noodles, and herbs on the bottom third of the rice paper. Fold both sides toward the center and roll the wrapper from bottom to top.

6. Soak and fill the remaining wrappers, then serve them with the dip.

Health Tip

These summer rolls are pure health food. Here's a short list of their most valuable components: fiber, potassium, and vitamin B_5, which are important for heart function since they lower both cholesterol and blood pressure; biotin, which is important for regulating blood sugar and is considered a "beauty vitamin" because of its positive effects on the skin; iron, a crucial element for red blood cells, which transport oxygen throughout the body; magnesium and manganese, both of which are responsible for sufficient energy production, muscle growth, and a stable nervous system; and vitamin K, which ensures stable bones and is necessary for blood coagulation. And that's only the short list!

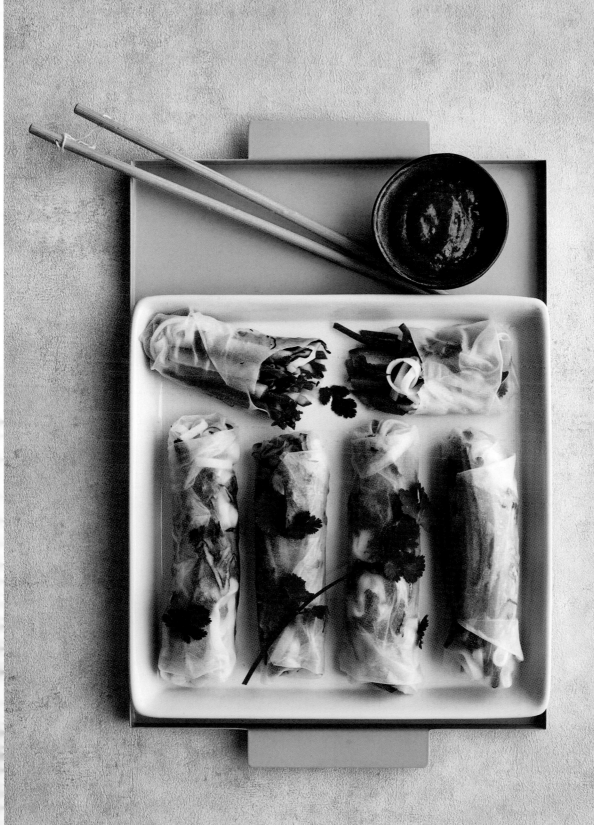

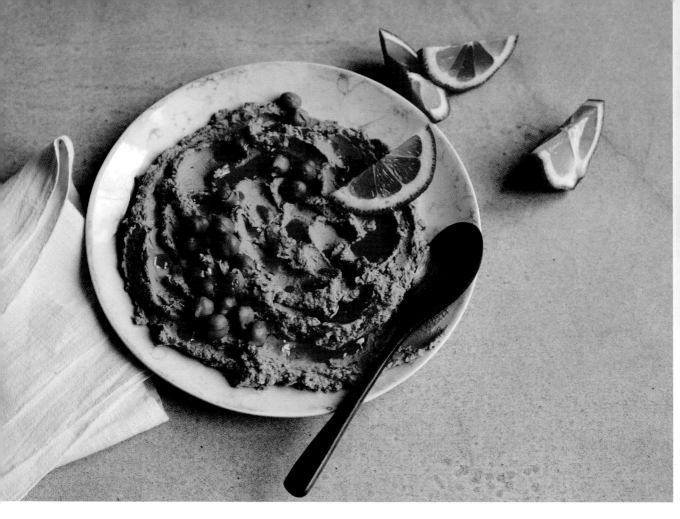

Classic Hummus

SERVES 2
PREP TIME: 10 minutes
PER SERVING: 315 calories, 10 g protein,
20 g fat, 18 g carbohydrates

2 tablespoons olive oil

2 tablespoons tahini

1¾ cups (340 g) drained, rinsed canned
  chickpeas

Juice of 1 lemon

1 tablespoon ground cumin

1. Blend the oil and tahini in a blender for
a few minutes, until smooth.

2. Add the chickpeas, lemon juice, and
cumin and blend for about 4 minutes,
until creamy. If necessary, add a teaspoon
or two of water. Pour into a bowl and serve.

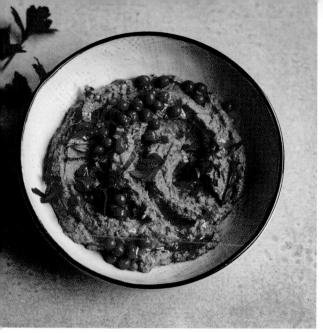

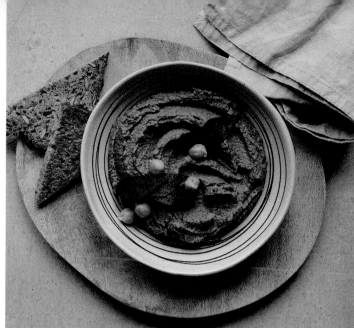

Green Pea Hummus

SERVES 2
PREP TIME: 10 minutes
PER SERVING: 385 calories, 15 g protein,
23 g fat, 29 g carbohydrates

½ bunch parsley
2 tablespoons olive oil
2 tablespoons tahini
1¾ cups (340 g) drained, rinsed canned
   chickpeas
1 cup (160 g) shelled fresh peas
Juice of 1 lemon
1 tablespoon ground cumin

1. Roughly chop the parsley.

2. Blend the oil and tahini in a blender for
a few minutes, until creamy.

3. Add the chickpeas, peas, lemon juice,
cumin, and parsley and blend for about 4
minutes, until creamy. If necessary, add a
teaspoon or two of water. Pour into a bowl
and serve.

Beet Hummus

SERVES 2
PREP TIME: 10 minutes
PER SERVING: 375 calories, 9 g protein,
22 g fat, 34 g carbohydrates

2 tablespoons olive oil
2 tablespoons tahini
2 cups (340 g) sliced cooked beets
1¾ cups (340 g) drained, rinsed canned
   chickpeas
Juice of 1 lemon
1 tablespoon ground cumin
Chili paste, to taste

1. Blend the oil and tahini in a blender for
a few minutes, until creamy.

2. Add the beets, chickpeas, lemon juice,
cumin, and chili paste, if desired, and
blend for about 4 minutes, until creamy. If
necessary, add a teaspoon or two of water.
Pour into a bowl and serve.

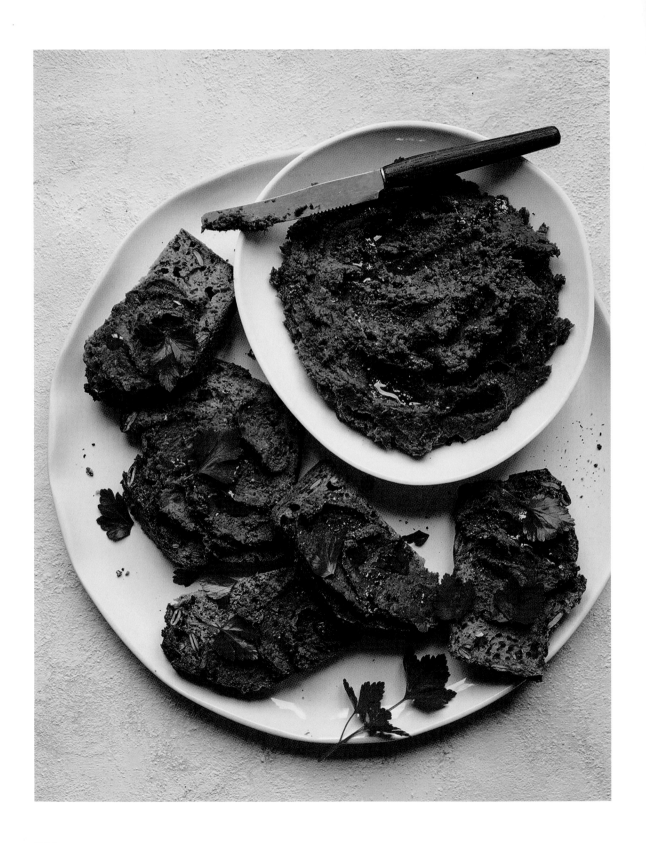

Tomato-Lentil Tapenade

SERVES 4
PREP TIME: 30 minutes
PER SERVING: 375 calories, 18 g protein, 12 g fat, 44 g carbohydrates

---

1½ cups (300 g) brown lentils
⅓ cup (40 g) dry-packed sun-dried tomatoes
1 onion
2 garlic cloves
¼ cup (60 ml) olive oil
1 tablespoon dried thyme
1 teaspoon sea salt

---

1. Rinse the lentils and cook according to the package instructions.

2. Meanwhile, place the tomatoes in a small bowl, pour boiling water over them, and soak for 15 minutes. Drain and press out any remaining water.

3. Peel the onion and garlic and dice.

4. Heat the oil in a skillet over medium-high heat and sauté the onion, garlic, and thyme for 3 minutes. Remove from the heat.

5. Drain the lentils. Transfer to a blender along with the onion mixture and tomatoes and blend until smooth.

6. Season with the salt, then pour into a bowl and serve.

NOTE: This spread goes well with our Pumpkin Seed and Chia Bread (page 158).

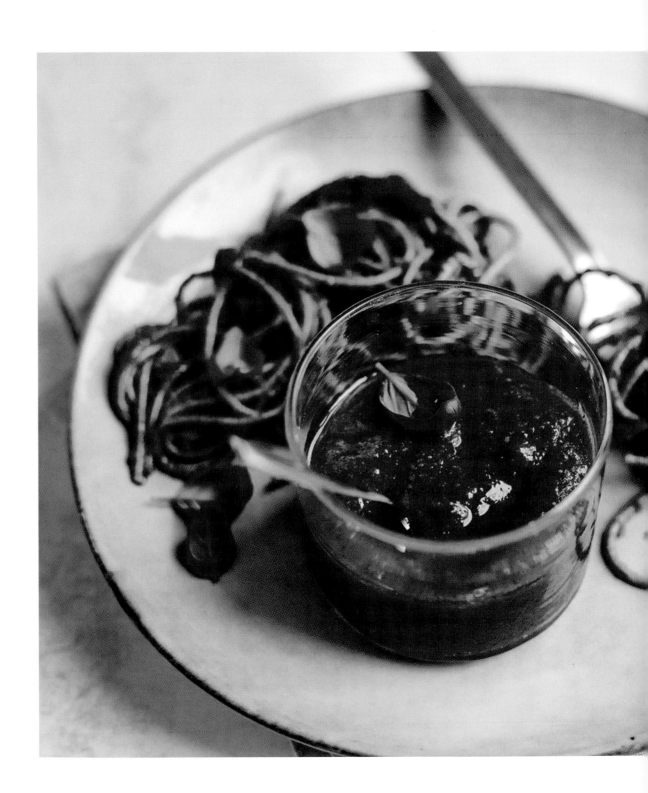

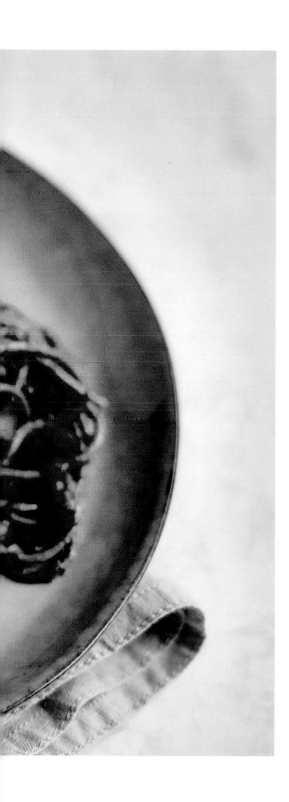

Basil Pesto

MAKES 1 SCANT CUP (200 G)
PREP TIME: 10 minutes
PER SERVING (1 TABLESPOON):
201 calories, 3 g protein, 21 g fat,
4 g carbohydrates

---

4 cups (100 g) fresh basil leaves
1 cup (100 g) raw walnuts
¾ cup (100 g) toasted pine nuts
Scant ⅔ cup (150 ml) olive oil, plus extra
   to top up the jar
1 peeled garlic clove
1 teaspoon sea salt

---

1. Blend all the ingredients in a food processor for a few minutes, until creamy. If the mixture is too solid, add some more oil.

2. Spoon into a clean jar and completely cover the surface with more oil. Serve and enjoy.

NOTE: Covered in olive oil and sealed airtight, this pesto can be kept in the refrigerator for at least 3 weeks. It is a tasty treat on pasta and potatoes, as a spread on bread, in a salad dressing, or as a dip with raw foods.

Vegetable Pasta with Avocado Sauce

SERVES 2
PREP TIME: 30 minutes
PER SERVING: 815 calories, 23 g protein, 37 g fat, 96 g carbohydrates

---

1 red onion
1 garlic clove
1 carrot
1 zucchini
2 tomatoes
7 ounces (200 g) whole wheat penne
Sea salt
2 tablespoons canola oil
1 teaspoon dried oregano
Red pepper flakes, optional
1 avocado
Juice of ½ lemon
Fresh ground black pepper

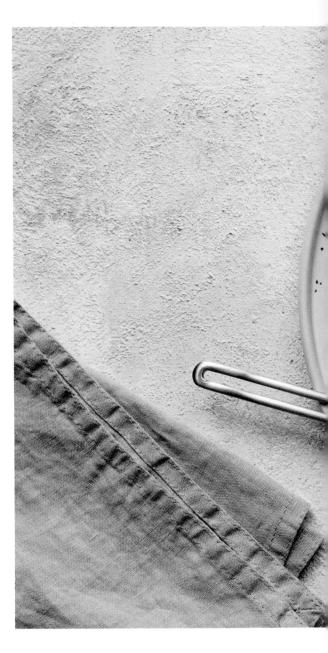

1. Peel and finely chop the onion and garlic. Finely dice the carrot, zucchini, and tomatoes.

2. Cook the penne in plenty of salted water according to the package instructions.

3. Meanwhile, heat the oil in a skillet over medium-high heat and sauté the onion and garlic for about 3 minutes, until soft. Add the carrot, zucchini, and tomatoes and sauté for another 5 minutes.

4. Season with the oregano and red pepper flakes, if using, and sauté for 2 more minutes.

5. Drain the penne, then add to the vegetables and stir to combine.

6. Halve, pit, and peel the avocado. Mash with a fork in a small bowl and mix with the lemon juice until it forms a creamy sauce. Season with salt and pepper and spoon it over the penne. Divide between bowls and serve.

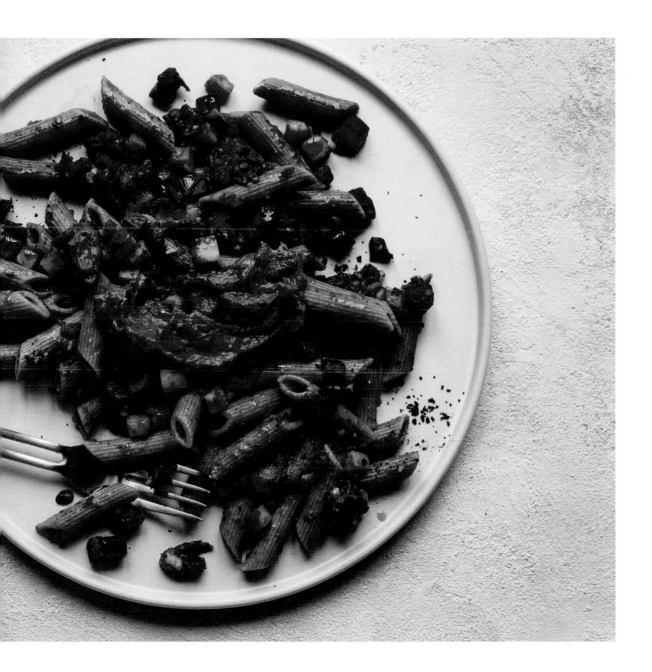

Health Tip

Whole wheat noodles are made from the complete grain, whereas "white" pasta consists mainly of wheat flour or durum wheat semolina. Whole wheat products retain the outer layers of the grain, including the germ—and that's where most of the fiber, minerals, vitamins, and healthy fats are found. Because whole wheat pasta contains complex carbohydrates, blood sugar rises more slowly, limiting insulin discharge after the meal.

Garlic-Zucchini Spaghetti

SERVES 2
PREP TIME: 20 minutes
PER SERVING: 660 calories, 19 g protein, 18 g fat, 99 g carbohydrates

9 ounces (250 g) spelt spaghetti
Sea salt
1 zucchini
3 garlic cloves
½ bunch parsley
1 tablespoon canola oil
2 tablespoons olive oil
3 teaspoons dried oregano
¼ cup (60 ml) white wine
Fresh ground black pepper

1. Cook the spaghetti in salted water according to the package instructions.

2. Meanwhile, dice the zucchini. Peel and thinly slice the garlic. Julienne the parsley.

3. Heat the canola oil in a skillet over medium heat and sauté the garlic for 1 minute, until fragrant. Add the olive oil, zucchini, and oregano and sauté for another 3 minutes. Deglaze with the wine.

4. Drain the spaghetti, then add to the pan with the zucchini and stir to combine. Season with salt and pepper.

5. Sprinkle with the parsley and serve immediately.

Health Tip

Spelt contains eight essential amino acids and more minerals than wheat— magnesium and iron, in particular. The silica found in spelt strengthens connective tissue and is important for maintaining healthy skin, strong fingernails, and shiny hair. Although spelt is a much older grain than wheat, it hasn't changed for hundreds of years, which is why many people today tolerate it better than wheat. But spelt is not completely gluten-free, making it unsuitable for people suffering from celiac disease. If you can't tolerate gluten, feel free to use gluten-free noodles for this recipe instead.

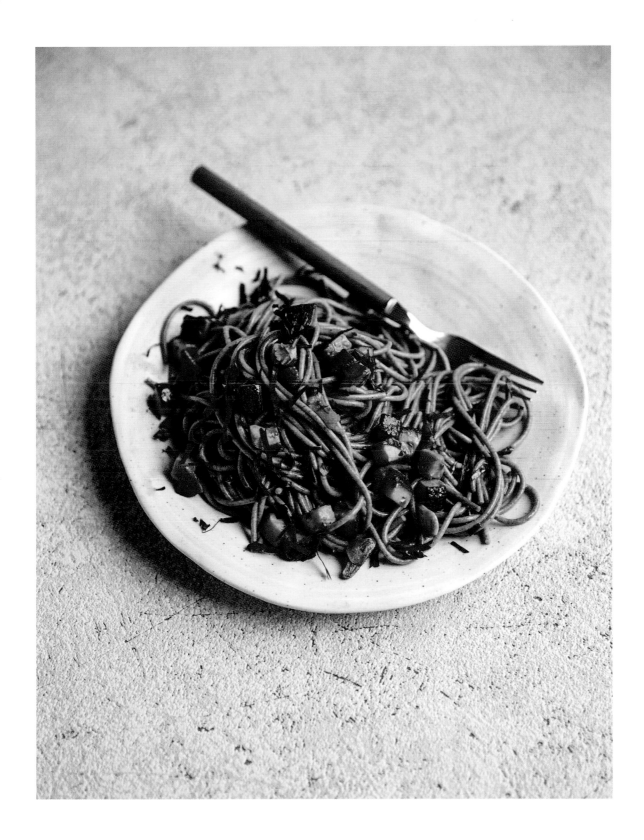

Butternut Squash Bake

SERVES 2
PREP TIME: 45 minutes
PER SERVING: 515 calories, 13 g protein,
45 g fat, 16 g carbohydrates

1½ cups (200 g) peeled, cubed butternut
  squash
1 scallion
2 handfuls watercress
¼ cup (40 g) pomegranate seeds
½ cup (60 g) pumpkin seeds

DRESSING
¼ cup (60 ml) pumpkin seed oil
¼ cup (60 ml) white wine vinegar
2 tablespoons Almond Butter (page 150)
Sea salt
Fresh ground black pepper

---

1. Preheat the oven to 350°F (180°C). Line a baking sheet with parchment paper.

2. Place the squash on the baking sheet. Bake for 30 minutes, then remove and let cool.

3. While the squash is in the oven, thinly slice the scallion.

4. To make the dressing, mix the oil, vinegar, and almond butter in a small bowl until creamy. Season with salt and pepper.

5. Divide the watercress between two bowls and top each with half of the butternut squash.

6. Pour on the dressing and toss to combine. Top with the scallions, pomegranate seeds, and pumpkin seeds, and serve.

Health Tip
Butternut squash is rich in beta carotene and important for maintaining healthy skin and hair. It also has very little fat and a ton healthy fiber and protein. Don't throw the seeds away! Rinse them in a bowl of water and then roast them in the oven at 350°F (180°C) for 20 minutes. They make a wonderful snack and can also be used as a topping for salads.

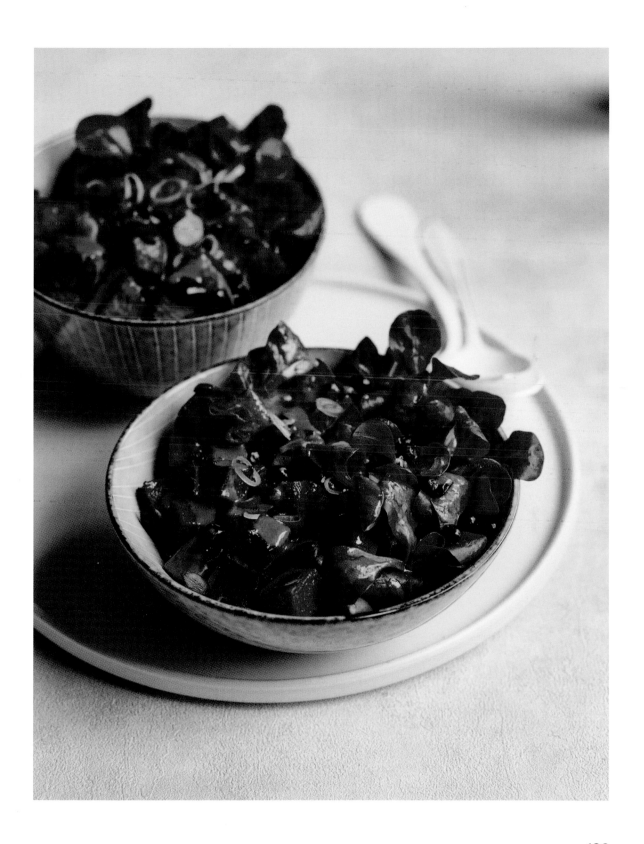

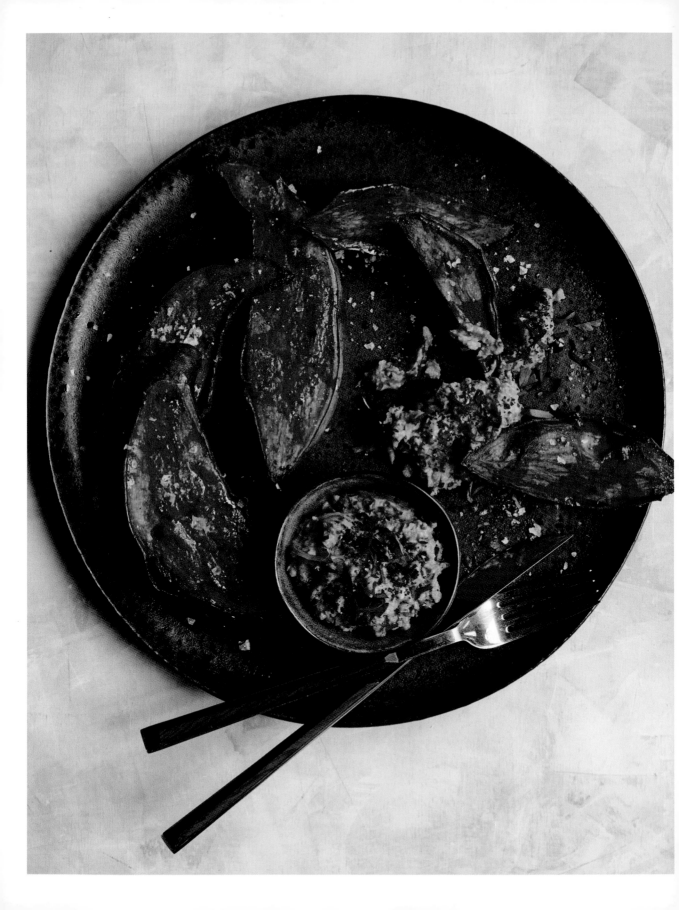

Baked Sweet Potato with Guacamole

SERVES 2
PREP TIME: 45 minutes
PER SERVING: 505 calories, 6 g protein, 33 g fat, 45 g carbohydrates

1 large sweet potato
1 tablespoon olive oil
Sea salt
Fresh ground black pepper
½ red onion
½ bunch cilantro
1 or 2 avocados
1 teaspoon ground cumin
2 tablespoons lemon juice
Red pepper flakes

1. Preheat the oven to 350°F (180°C). Line a baking sheet with parchment paper.

2. Cut the sweet potato into wedges. Transfer to the baking sheet, drizzle with the oil, and season with salt and pepper. Bake for 30 minutes, or until tender. Remove and let cool.

3. Meanwhile, peel and finely dice the onion. Julienne the cilantro.

4. Halve, pit, and peel the avocado, then mash with a fork in a medium bowl. Add the onion, cilantro, cumin, and lemon juice and mix until creamy. Season with salt, pepper, and red pepper flakes.

5. Arrange the sweet potato wedges on plates and serve with the guacamole.

Health Tip

Sweet potatoes contain lots of beta carotene, which is good for the eyes and for maintaining healthy skin. Their many secondary phytochemicals make them true antiaging agents and protect us against any number of lifestyle diseases. Try to purchase only organic sweet potatoes and be sure to eat the skin, since that's where the secondary phytochemicals reside. These are particularly effective against anemia, high blood pressure, and diabetes.

Red Squash and Fennel Stew

SERVES 2
PREP TIME: 30 minutes
PER SERVING: 395 calories, 14 g protein, 14 g fat, 58 g carbohydrates

---

1 red onion
1 garlic clove
1 fennel bulb
1 red bell pepper
2 tablespoons coconut oil
1 tablespoon Vegetable Broth Paste (page 174)
1 teaspoon cayenne pepper
3½ cups (450 g) cubed red kuri or butternut squash
1¾ cups (200 g) drained, rinsed canned chickpeas
One 14.5-ounce (411 g) can whole peeled tomatoes
2 teaspoons fennel seeds

1. Peel and finely chop the onion and garlic. Chop the fennel and bell pepper into bite-size pieces.

2. Heat the oil in a large pot over medium heat. Add the broth paste, onion, garlic, and cayenne and sauté for a few minutes, until softened.

3. Add the squash, chickpeas, fennel, and bell pepper and mix well. Stir in the tomatoes and a scant ½ cup (100 ml) water. Bring to a boil, then simmer over low heat for 10 minutes.

4. Divide between two bowls. Sprinkle with the fennel seeds and serve.

> Health Tip
> Whether eaten raw or cooked, as a tea or as a spice, fennel is always a good thing. It has a calming effect on the stomach and the entire digestive system. In fact, it's very effective against bloating and constipation. Fennel also has a cleansing effect: It helps to rid the body of superfluous fluids via the urinary system. All in all, it's an excellent detox vegetable that deserves to find its way onto your plate.

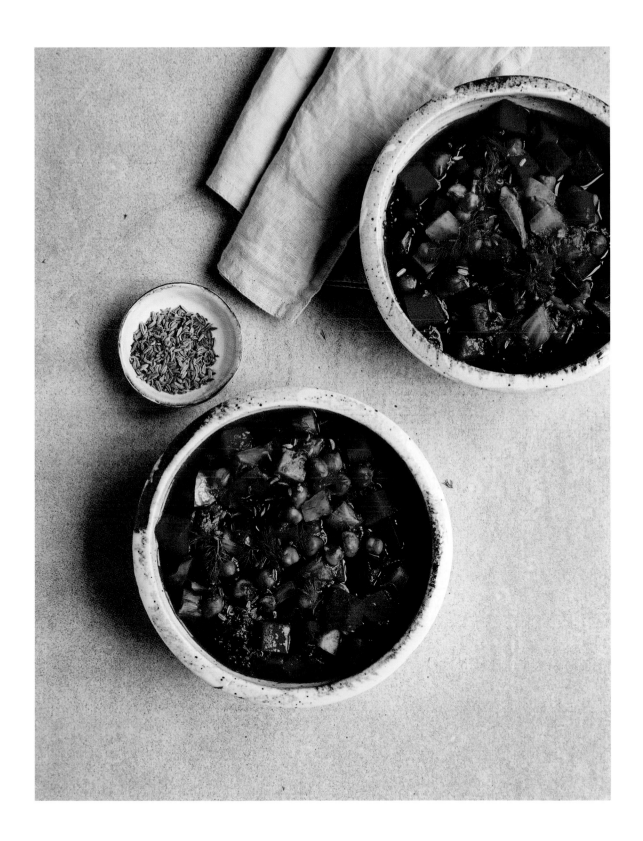

Potato-Mushroom Stew

SERVES 2
PREP TIME: 45 minutes
PER SERVING: 465 calories, 13 g protein,
21 g fat, 45 g carbohydrates

---

7 ounces (200 g) button mushrooms
7 ounces (200 g) king oyster mushrooms
2 carrots
1 celery rib
1 red onion
2 garlic cloves
¼ cup (60 ml) canola oil
2 tablespoons tomato paste
4 medium potatoes
Scant ½ cup (100 ml) red wine
1 teaspoon Vegetable Broth Paste
  (page 174)
1 teaspoon dried thyme
1 bay leaf
1 tablespoon maple syrup
Sea salt
Fresh ground black pepper
½ bunch parsley

---

1. Quarter the button mushrooms and halve the oyster mushrooms. Slice the carrots and celery. Peel and finely dice the onion and garlic.

2. Heat half of the oil in a large pot over medium heat and sauté the garlic and mushrooms for 5 minutes. Remove from the heat and set aside.

3. Heat the remaining oil in a skillet over medium heat and sauté the onions, carrots, and celery for 3 minutes, until soft. Add the tomato paste and cook for 3 more minutes, stirring constantly.

4. Peel and dice the potatoes, then add to the mushrooms in the pot. Add the vegetables from the skillet and cook over medium heat, stirring to combine.

5. Deglaze with the wine and scant 1 cup (200 ml) water.

6. Add the thyme, bay leaf, and maple syrup, and season with salt and pepper. Cover and simmer over low heat for 20 minutes. Stir occasionally.

7. Julienne the parsley. Divide the stew between two bowls, remove the bay leaf, sprinkle with parsley, and serve.

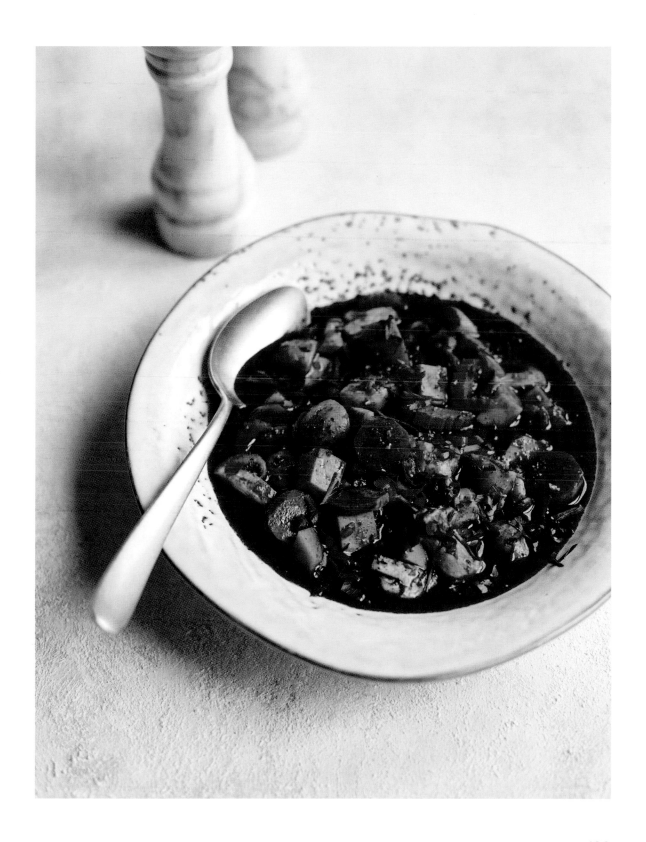

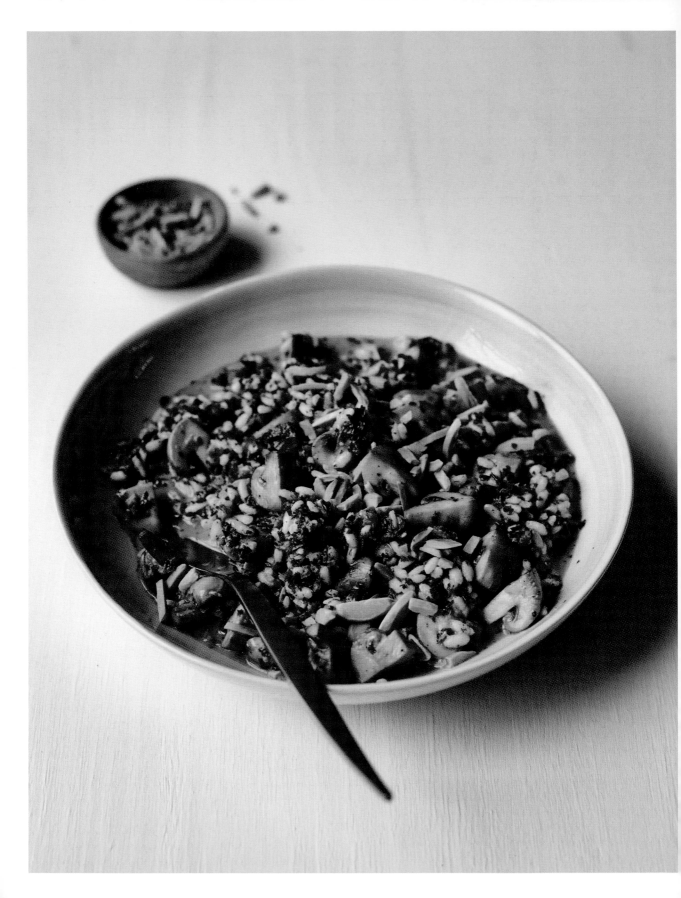

Coconut-Kale Risotto

SERVES 2
PREP TIME: 45 minutes
PER SERVING: 765 calories, 25 g protein, 30 g fat, 88 g carbohydrates

---

9 ounces (250 g) mushrooms
1 red onion
2 garlic cloves
1 tablespoon coconut oil
1 cup (200 g) Arborio or carnaroli rice
3 tablespoons Vegetable Broth Paste (page 174)
Scant ½ cup (100 ml) white wine
3 cups (300 g) kale leaves
Scant ½ cup (100 ml) coconut milk
Sea salt
Fresh ground black pepper
½ cup (50 g) slivered almonds

---

1. Clean and quarter the mushrooms. Peel and finely chop the onion and garlic.

2. Heat the oil in a pot over medium-high heat. Sauté the mushrooms, onion, and garlic until the onions are translucent, about 5 minutes, stirring constantly.

3. Rinse and drain the rice. Add to the pot along with the vegetable broth paste and sauté for 2 minutes.

4. Deglaze with the wine, then add 2½ cups (600 ml) water.

5. Let the rice simmer half-covered over low heat for 20 minutes, stirring regularly.

6. While the rice cooks, stem and finely chop the kale.

7. Add the kale and coconut milk to the pot and mix well. Simmer for another 10 minutes, stirring regularly.

8. Season with salt and pepper. Divide between two bowls, top with the almonds, and serve.

NOTE: In the spring, try this risotto with asparagus. Wash 10½ ounces (300 g) asparagus and cut off the tough ends. Cook the asparagus in boiling salted water for 5 minutes until al dente, drain, and mix into the rice.

Mediterranean Tomato-Bean Sauté

SERVES 2
PREP TIME: 20 minutes
PER SERVING: 215 calories, 11 g protein,
6 g fat, 28 g carbohydrates

---

14 ounces (400 g) tomatoes

5 scallions

1 tablespoon coconut oil

1 teaspoon dried thyme

1 tablespoon dried rosemary

3 cups (300 g) trimmed, chopped green
beans

½ cup (150 g) drained, rinsed canned
kidney beans

Sea salt

Fresh ground black pepper

---

1. Dice the tomatoes and thinly slice the scallions.

2. Heat the oil in a large skillet over medium heat, add the thyme and rosemary, and sauté for 1 minute, stirring constantly.

3. Add the tomatoes, scallions, and green beans and cook for another 5 minutes.

4. Add the kidney beans and simmer for 2 minutes, then season with salt and pepper. Divide between bowls and serve.

Health Tip

Tomatoes originate from South America. Today, we know of over 2,500 different types, all of which contain high levels of vitamin C, many B vitamins, iron, and folic acid. One of the most important health advantages of tomatoes lies in the pigment lycopene, which neutralizes free radicals, protects skin from dangerous UV light, helps to reduce damaging deposits in blood vessels, and stops the production of cancer cells. To get the full benefits of the lycopene, the tomatoes must first be cooked.

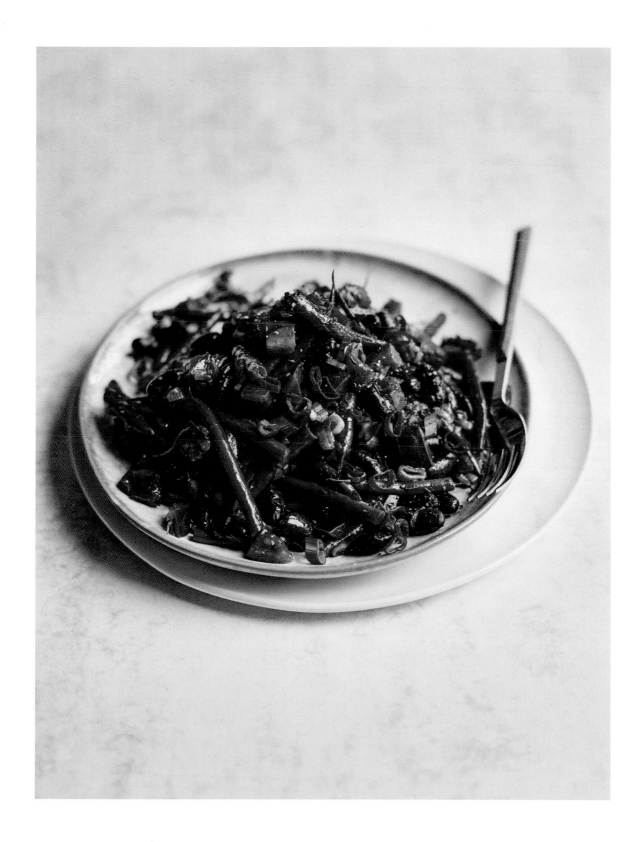

Rainbow Roasted
Root Vegetables

SERVES 2
PREP TIME: 45 minutes
PER SERVING: 420 calories, 8 g protein,
12 g fat, 70 g carbohydrates

---

2 purple carrots
2 orange carrots
1 fennel bulb
2 small parsnips
1 beet
1 large sweet potato
2 tablespoons olive oil
2 rosemary sprigs
3 thyme sprigs
Sea salt
Fresh ground black pepper

---

1. Preheat the oven to 350°F (180°C). Line a baking sheet with parchment paper.

2. Cut the carrots, fennel, parsnips, beet, and sweet potato into large pieces or wedges. Place on the baking sheet and drizzle with the oil. Sprinkle on the thyme and rosemary sprigs. Season with salt and pepper.

3. Bake for 30 minutes, or until tender. Divide between plates and serve alone, or with Classic Hummus (page 182) or Guacamole (page 105).

Health Tip

A long-overlooked vegetable, parsnips are one of the healthiest root vegetables around. They have a sweet-spicy flavor, and because they contain a high concentration of carbohydrates, they are very filling. Harvested and eaten in the fall or winter, parsnips are rich in vitamin C and potassium and thus important for building muscles. But they are especially valuable because of their high fiber content, which is broken down in the intestinal tract by bacteria and then swells up when it comes into contact with fluids, revving up intestinal peristalsis.

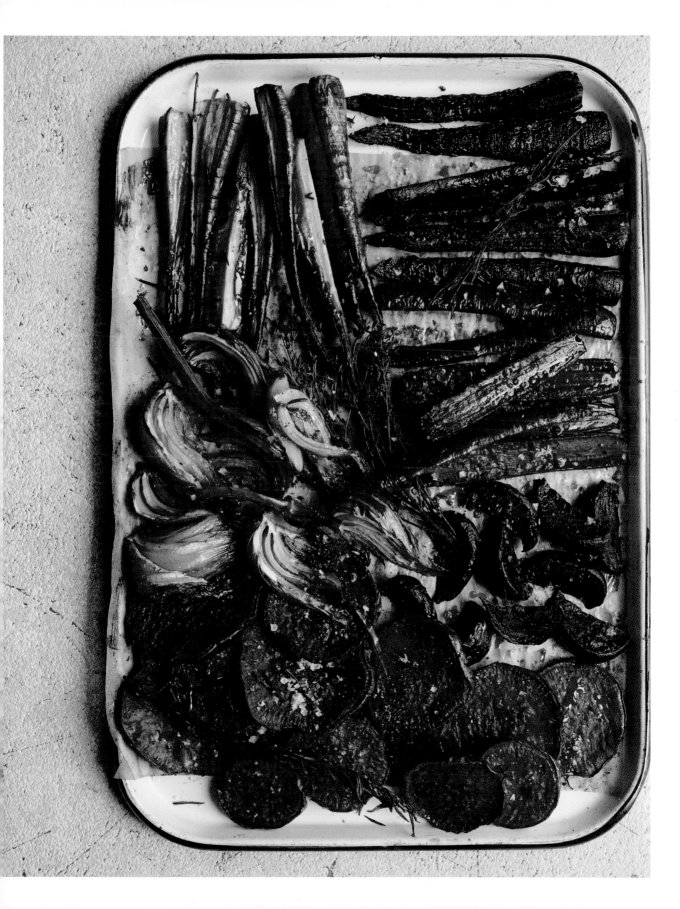

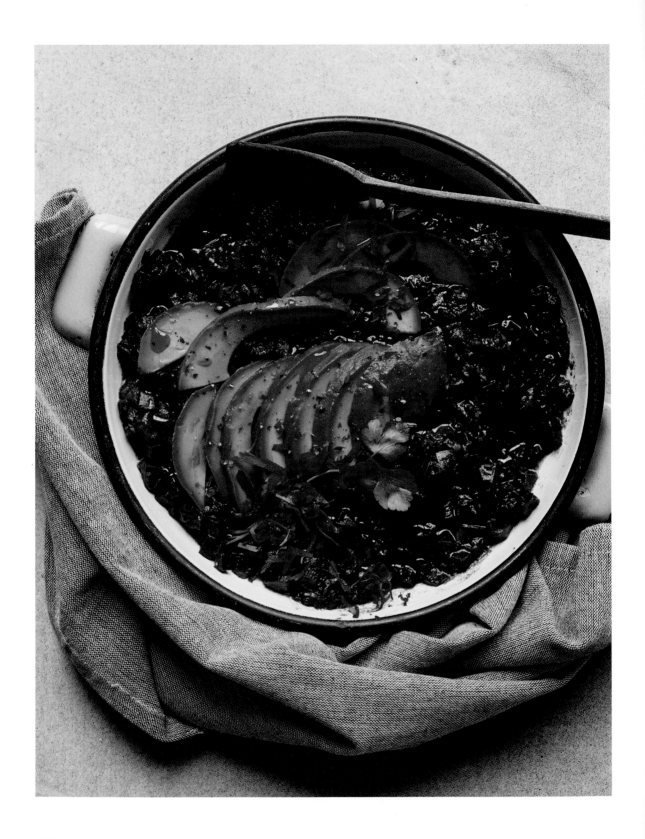

Shakshuka with Avocado

SERVES 2
PREP TIME: 40 minutes
PER SERVING: 405 calories, 7 g protein, 35 g fat, 15 g carbohydrates

---

2 red bell peppers
14 ounces (400 g) tomatoes
1 small red onion
2 garlic cloves
2 tablespoons canola oil
2 teaspoons ground cumin
2 tablespoons tomato paste
1 tablespoon harissa
Sea salt
Fresh ground black pepper
1 avocado
2 tablespoons chopped cilantro

---

1. Dice the bell peppers and tomatoes. Peel and finely chop the onion and garlic.

2. Heat the oil in a skillet over medium-high heat and add the onion, bell peppers, and cumin. Sauté for about 8 minutes, until softened, stirring occasionally.

3. Add the garlic, tomato paste, and harissa and sauté the mixture for another 2 minutes.

4. Add the tomatoes, season with salt and pepper, then bring to a simmer over medium-low heat for 15 to 20 minutes, stirring occasionally so the tomatoes don't burn.

5. Halve, pit, and peel the avocado, then dice or slice the flesh. Garnish the shakshuka with the avocado and cilantro and serve.

NOTES: This goes well with the Pumpkin Seed and Chia Bread (page 158).

Double the recipe so that, together with 1 cup (240 ml) water and 1 teaspoon Vegetable Broth Paste (page 174), you can blend half of it the next day in your mixer. Then heat it in a small pot: Now you have a tasty tomato soup!

Potato-Leek Soup

SERVES 2
PREP TIME: 30 minutes
PER SERVING: 235 calories, 9 g protein,
7 g fat, 32 g carbohydrates

2 leeks
3 medium potatoes
2 carrots
1 tablespoon Vegetable Broth Paste
  (page 174)
½ bunch parsley
Sea salt
Fresh ground black pepper
2 tablespoons vegan sour cream

1. Wash the leeks and slice into rings. Peel and dice the potatoes. Dice the carrots. Transfer to a large pot.

2. Add the broth paste and 2 cups (480 ml) water to the pot, bring to a boil, then turn the heat to low to simmer for 15 minutes, or until the vegetables have softened.

3. Meanwhile, julienne the parsley.

4. Blend the soup with an immersion blender until creamy and season with salt and pepper.

5. Stir in the sour cream. Divide the soup between two bowls, sprinkle with the parsley, and serve.

NOTE: You can modify the basic recipe by adding various other things, for example, diced potatoes fried in olive oil, croutons made from whole wheat bread, or fried mushrooms. For an extra portion of healthy fats and minerals, scatter some fried sunflower seeds or chopped hazelnuts into the soup.

Health Tip
Leeks contain a ton of iron, potassium, and vitamin C to get your metabolism going. They are also anti-inflammatory. Potatoes are a good source of protein, since our body can easily use their amino acids.

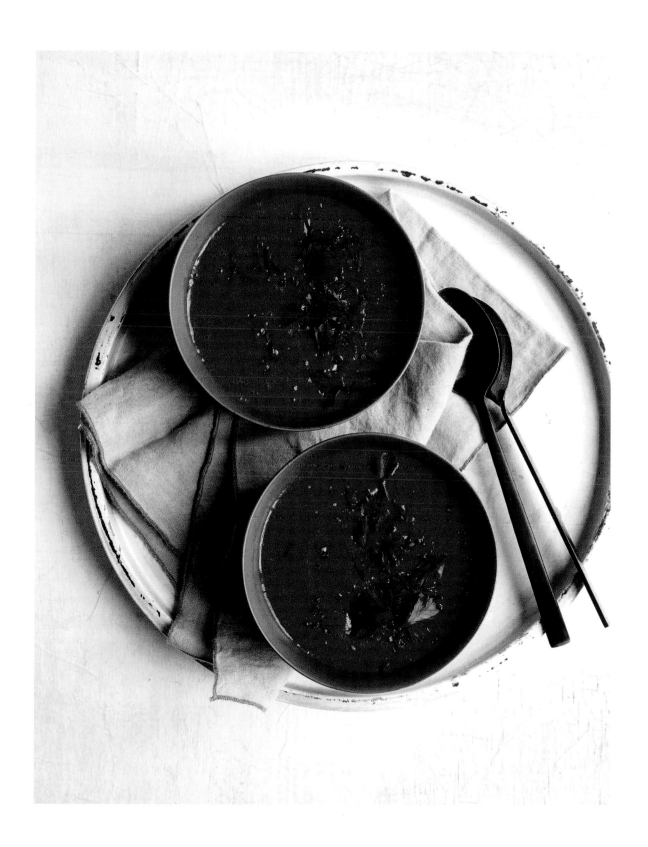

Thai Coconut Noodle Soup

SERVES 2
PREP TIME: 45 minutes
PER SERVING: 720 calories, 20 g protein, 41 g fat, 62 g carbohydrates

---

3½ ounces (100 g) rice noodles
⅓ cup (50 g) cashews
2 garlic cloves
1-inch (2.5 cm) piece ginger
½ bunch cilantro
1 teaspoon chili paste
Juice of 1 lime
1 cup (240 ml) coconut milk
3 tablespoons soy sauce
Sea salt
Fresh ground black pepper
2 tablespoons Vegetable Broth Paste
    (page 174)
1 handful cremini mushrooms
1 carrot
5 cups (100 g) baby spinach
½ bunch Thai basil
1 cup (100 g) bean sprouts
½ lime, cut into wedges
1 tablespoon chili oil

---

1. Cook the noodles according to the package instructions, rinse with cold water, and set aside.

2. Toast the cashews in a dry skillet over medium heat for about 5 minutes, until fragrant. Peel and finely dice the garlic and ginger.

3. Transfer the cashews, garlic, and ginger to a blender with the cilantro, chili paste, lime juice, coconut milk, and soy sauce and blend into a smooth paste. Season with salt and pepper.

4. Combine the broth paste with 3 cups (750 ml) water in a large pot and bring to a boil. Add the cashew paste, bring to a boil once more, turn the heat to low, and simmer for 10 minutes.

5. Meanwhile, clean and quarter the mushrooms and slice the carrot at an angle.

6. Add to the pot and simmer for 10 minutes. Add the spinach and simmer for another 5 minutes, until the spinach has wilted and the liquid has reduced slightly.

7. Divide the noodles between two bowls and ladle the soup on top. Garnish with the basil leaves, bean sprouts, and lime wedges. Drizzle with the chili oil and serve.

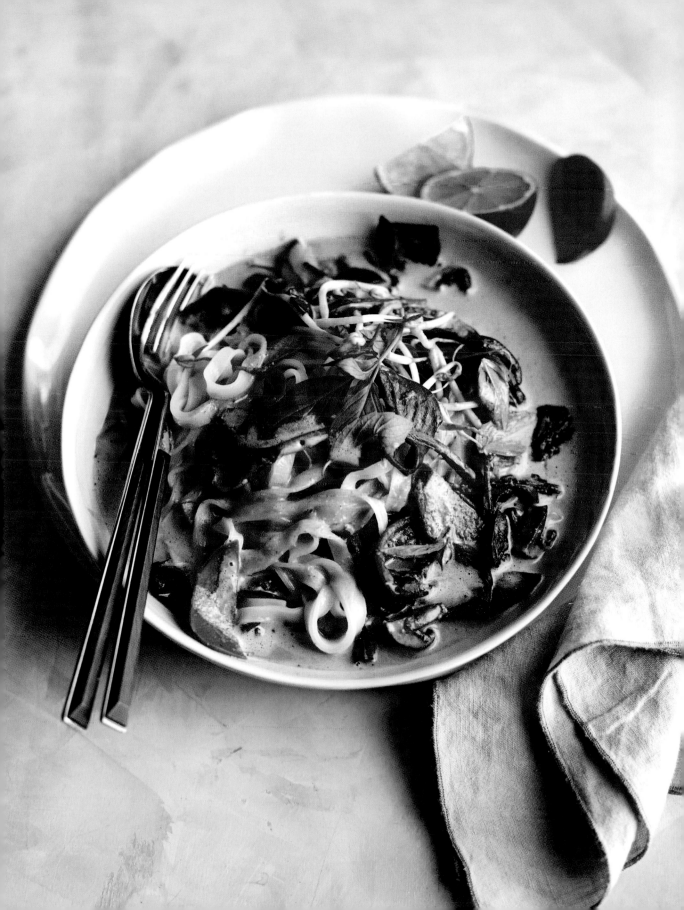

Dinner

Frisée Salad with Kidney Beans and Sprouts

SERVES 2
PREP TIME: 20 minutes
PER SERVING: 600 calories, 16 g protein, 45 g fat, 30 g carbohydrates

---

½ head frisée
½ head radicchio
1 small cucumber
¾ cup (180 g) drained, rinsed canned kidney beans
1 handful alfalfa sprouts
1 avocado

DRESSING
¼ cup (60 ml) olive oil
3 tablespoons apple cider vinegar
Juice of ½ lemon
1 tablespoon Dijon mustard
1 garlic clove
Sea salt
Fresh ground black pepper

---

1. Tear the frisée and radicchio into bite-size pieces into two bowls. Dice the cucumber and add to the bowls along with the kidney beans.

2. Rinse the sprouts in a sieve and let drain. Halve, pit, peel, and slice the avocado.

3. To make the dressing, mix the oil, vinegar, lemon juice, and Dijon mustard in a small bowl until creamy. Peel and press the garlic and add it to the dressing. Season with salt and pepper.

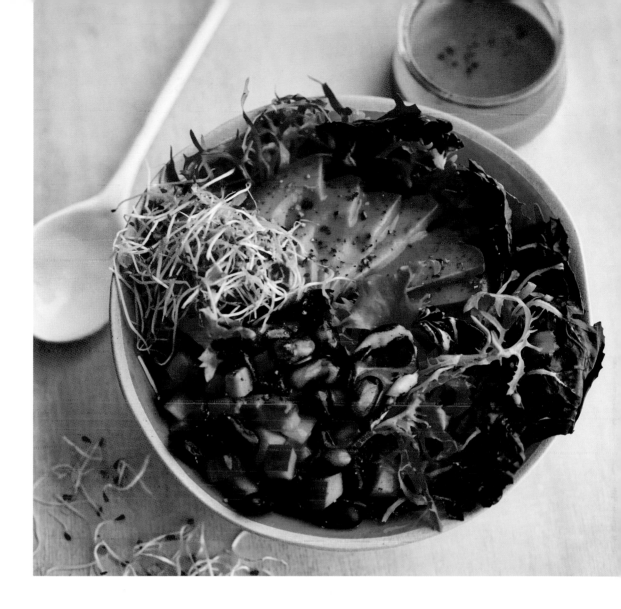

4. Pour the dressing into the bowls and toss. Top with the avocado and sprouts and serve.

NOTE: Instead of using an avocado for the topping, you can sprinkle on some chopped walnuts.

Health Tip

Frisée is a summer lettuce with a slightly bitter taste to it. But it's these bitter compounds that help our body to detox, by supporting the kidneys, liver, and gallbladder. Kidney beans are a valuable source of plant protein and fiber and are rich in magnesium (140 milligrams per 100 grams beans)—the ideal fitness food, since this mineral prevents cramps and muscle aches.

Chickpea Protein Bowl

SERVES 2
PREP TIME: 20 minutes
PER SERVING: 670 calories, 13 g protein, 59 g fat, 19 g carbohydrates

---

Sea salt
3½ ounces (100 g) green beans
3 scallions
½ cup (50 g) walnuts
1 cup (200 g) drained, rinsed canned chickpeas
3 cups (100 g) watercress

DRESSING
¼ cup (60 ml) avocado oil
2 tablespoons balsamic vinegar
1 teaspoon ground cumin
1 garlic clove
Sea salt
Fresh ground black pepper

---

1. Bring a pot of salted water to a boil and blanch the green beans until bright green and tender-crisp, about 3 to 5 minutes. Drain, then plunge immediately into an ice-water bath to stop the cooking. Drain and set aside.

2. Thinly slice the scallions. Coarsely chop the walnuts.

3. To make the dressing, mix the oil with the vinegar and cumin in a small bowl. Peel, press, and add the garlic. Season with salt and pepper.

4. Combine the green beans, chickpeas, and scallions in a medium bowl with the dressing. Top with the watercress and walnuts and serve.

Health Tip
Like all legumes, chickpeas are true protein bombs: 3½ ounces (100 grams) chickpeas have 20 grams protein and the essential amino acids lysine and threonine, which our body cannot produce on its own. Furthermore, a single portion contains nearly three fourths of the daily recommended dose of folic acid, one fourth of the daily dose of iron, and one fifth of our daily zinc needs. Chickpeas also have lots of fiber to keep your digestion going and the lining of your intestinal system healthy. This in turn prevents diseases of the colon, such as colon cancer. The high level of vitamin E makes chickpeas the perfect antiaging food. But we also love chickpeas because there are just so many excellent ways to prepare them.

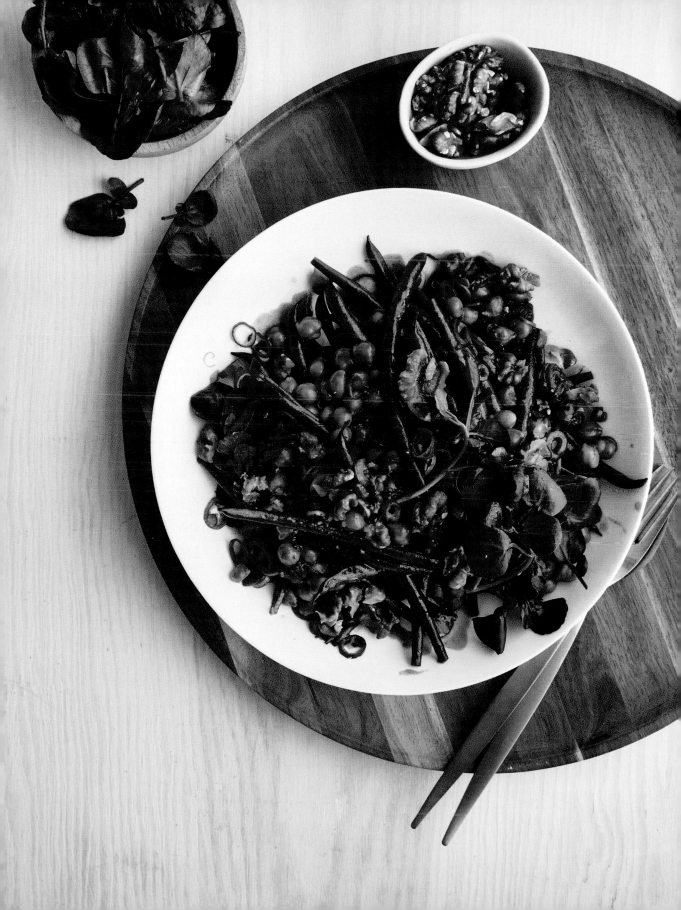

Potato and Green Bean Salad with Smoked Tofu

SERVES 2
PREP TIME: 40 minutes
PER SERVING: 720 calories, 27 g protein, 40 g fat, 62 g carbohydrates

---

Sea salt
6 medium potatoes
2 scallions
2 tomatoes
7 ounces (200 g) smoked tofu
2 tablespoons canola oil
10½ ounces (300 g) green beans
4 large pickled cucumbers

DRESSING
¼ cup (60 ml) lemon juice
¼ cup (60 ml) olive oil
¼ cup (60 ml) apple cider vinegar
1 tablespoon coconut sugar
Sea salt
Fresh ground black pepper

---

1. Bring a pot of salted water to a boil, add the potatoes, and cook for 20 minutes, or until fork tender. Drain and let cool. Peel and cut into slices (about ½ inch/1 cm thick), then transfer to a large bowl.

2. Thinly slice the scallions and dice the tomatoes and tofu.

3. Heat the canola oil in a skillet over high heat and add the scallions, green beans, and tofu. Cook for about 5 minutes, until the vegetables have softened and the tofu is slightly golden brown. Remove from the heat and transfer to the bowl with the potatoes.

4. Slice the pickles and add to the bowl.

5. To make the dressing, combine the lemon juice, oil, vinegar, and sugar in a small bowl and season with salt and pepper.

6. Pour the dressing over the salad and toss to combine. Divide between two bowls and enjoy.

NOTE: For salads, we prefer smoked tofu, which is more flavorful than the "classic" white type. If you like things a little spicier, place the tofu in a mixture of oil and spices or a soy sauce marinade for 1 to 3 hours before dicing.

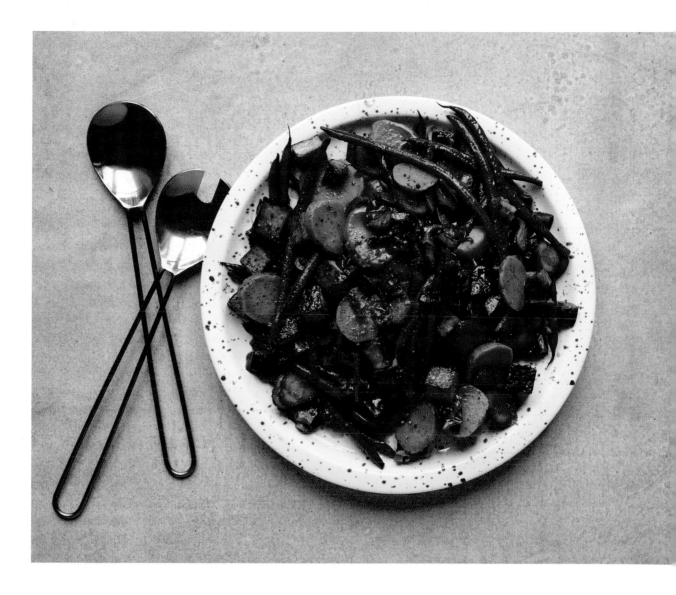

Health Tip

What makes tofu so valuable for vegetarians and vegans? Our body can easily turn the protein in tofu into our own protein components. In addition, tofu is cholesterol-free, which can help to lower your cholesterol level. It also contains phytoestrogens, which have a positive effect on our hormone balance as well as an apparent preventive effect on breast cancer, ovarian cancer, and cervical cancer.

Cauliflower Curry with Pearl Barley

SERVES 2
PREP TIME: 50 minutes
PER SERVING: 595 calories, 20 g protein, 26 g fat, 67 g carbohydrates

⅓ cup (80 g) pearl barley
1 handful cashews
½ head cauliflower
2 medium potatoes
1 red onion
1 garlic clove
1-inch (2.5 cm) piece ginger
2 tablespoons coconut oil
1 teaspoon garam masala
1 teaspoon ground turmeric
1 teaspoon ground coriander
1 cup (200 g) chopped tomatoes
1 tablespoon tomato paste
Sea salt
Fresh ground black pepper
3 tablespoons soy yogurt
Juice of 1 lemon
½ bunch cilantro
Red pepper flakes, optional

1. Cook the barley according to the package instructions.

2. Meanwhile, toast the cashews in a dry skillet over medium heat for about 3 minutes, until golden.

3. Cut the cauliflower into small florets. Peel and dice the potatoes. Peel and finely chop the onions, garlic, and ginger.

4. Heat the oil in a large pot over high heat and add the onion, garlic, and ginger. Cook for 3 minutes, or until softened, then add the garam masala, turmeric, and coriander.

5. Add the potatoes and cauliflower and cook for another 5 minutes, stirring often.

6. Add the tomatoes to the pot along with the tomato paste and scant ½ cup (100 ml) water. Season with salt and pepper, then cover and simmer over low heat for 15 minutes.

7. Combine the yogurt and lemon juice in a small bowl. Finely chop and add the cilantro. Stir in the red pepper flakes, if using.

8. Arrange the cauliflower curry and the barley in two bowls, top with the yogurt mixture and cashews, and serve.

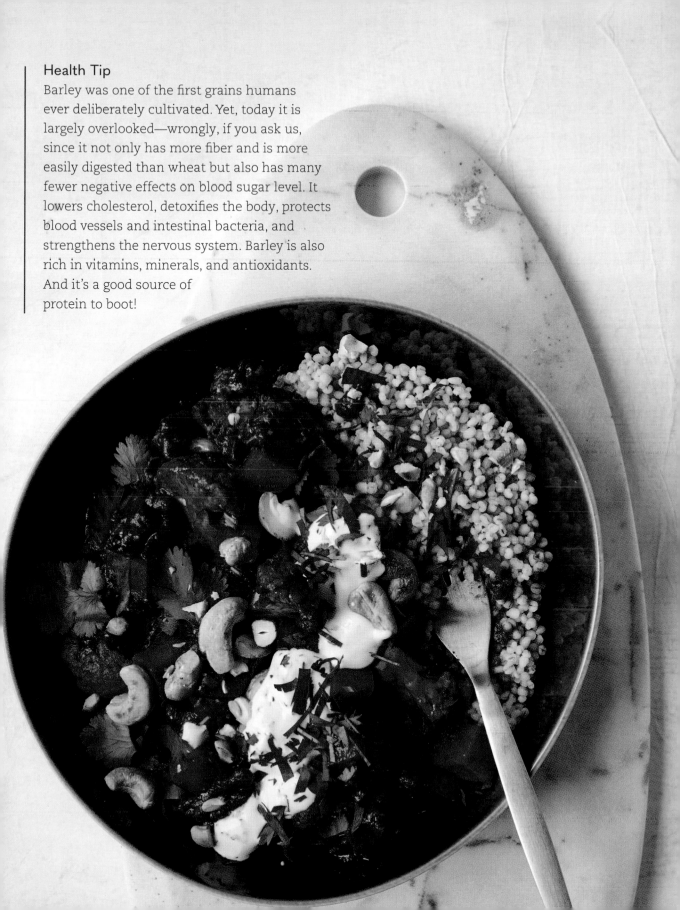

Health Tip

Barley was one of the first grains humans ever deliberately cultivated. Yet, today it is largely overlooked—wrongly, if you ask us, since it not only has more fiber and is more easily digested than wheat but also has many fewer negative effects on blood sugar level. It lowers cholesterol, detoxifies the body, protects blood vessels and intestinal bacteria, and strengthens the nervous system. Barley is also rich in vitamins, minerals, and antioxidants. And it's a good source of protein to boot!

Escarole Salad with Fava Beans

SERVES 2
PREP TIME: 20 minutes
PER SERVING: 330 calories, 10 g protein, 21 g fat, 24 g carbohydrates

---

2 carrots
1 red bell pepper
1 handful sugar snap peas
2 handfuls escarole leaves
1 cup (200 g) drained, rinsed canned fava beans
2 tablespoons alfalfa sprouts

DRESSING
¼ cup (60 ml) olive oil
3 tablespoons fresh orange juice
2 tablespoons white wine vinegar
Sea salt
Fresh ground black pepper

---

1. Finely dice the carrots and bell pepper and thinly slice the sugar snap peas. Tear the escarole leaves into bite-size pieces. Transfer to a large bowl along with the beans.

2. To make the dressing, combine the oil, orange juice, and vinegar in a small bowl. Season with salt and pepper.

3. Pour the dressing over the salad and toss to combine. Divide between two bowls, top with the sprouts, and serve.

Health Tip
The light green leaves of the escarole contain a bunch of bitter compounds. Especially interesting is the substance lactucopicrin, which stimulates digestion, is a diuretic, and promotes detoxification. If, despite these advantages, it is still too bitter for you, soak the leaves in lukewarm water for a short time before preparing them. Escarole is rich in potassium, calcium, phosphates, and folic acid, besides also being an excellent source of beta carotene.

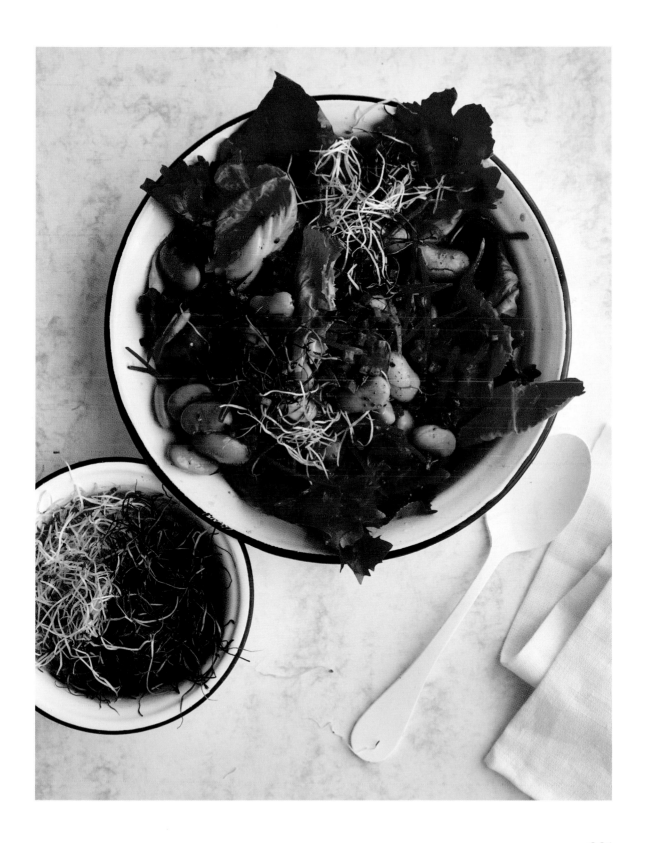

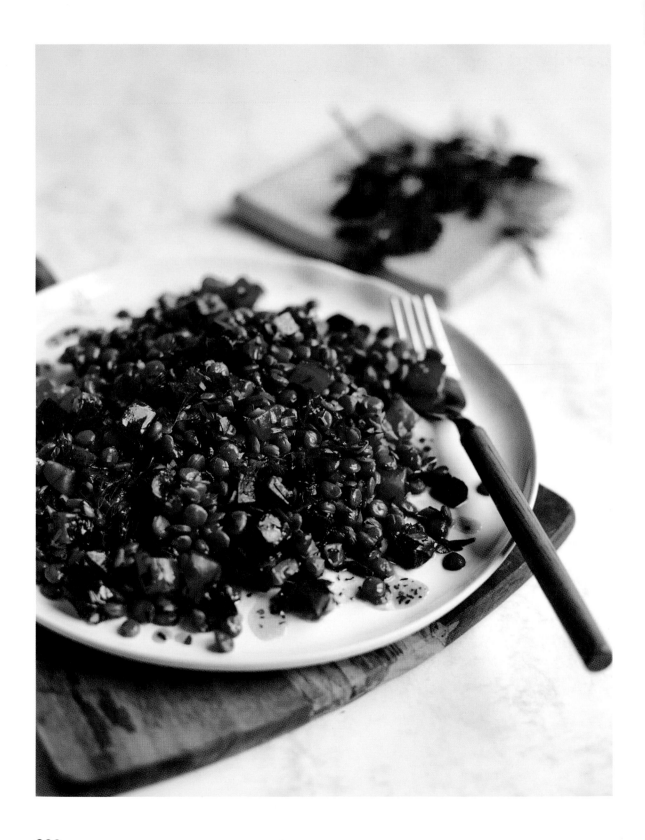

Lentil and Pepper Salad

SERVES 2
PREP TIME: 60 minutes
PER SERVING: 380 calories, 19 g protein, 11 g fat, 45 g carbohydrates

¾ cup (150 g) brown lentils
1 red bell pepper
1 yellow bell pepper
1 small red onion
½ bunch dill
½ bunch parsley

DRESSING
¼ cup (60 ml) olive oil
1 tablespoon white wine vinegar
2 teaspoons lemon juice
1 teaspoon dried marjoram
1 teaspoon dried thyme
Sea salt
Fresh ground black pepper

1. Rinse and drain the lentils, then cook according to the package instructions. Drain and set aside.

2. While the lentils cook, dice the bell peppers. Peel and finely dice the onion. Finely chop the dill and parsley.

3. To make the dressing, combine the oil, vinegar, lemon juice, marjoram, and thyme in a small bowl. Season with salt and pepper.

4. Transfer the lentils and vegetables to a medium bowl. Pour on the dressing and toss to combine. Divide between two bowls and serve.

NOTE: The flavors in this salad develop better if you first let it sit for a while before eating.

Health Tip
Lentils have little fat in them, but they've got lots of protein and high-quality carbohydrates. They're a perfect source of protein and energy for athletes. Their many B vitamins support brain function and strengthen the nervous system. They're also extremely filling due to their high level of fiber.

Broccoli Quinoa Bowl

SERVES 2
PREP TIME: 40 minutes
PER SERVING: 560 calories, 21 g protein, 33 g fat, 43 g carbohydrates

½ cup (90 g) quinoa

1 head broccoli

Sea salt

2 handfuls baby spinach

Scant 1 cup (170 g) drained, rinsed canned chickpeas

2 tablespoons slivered almonds

DRESSING

Juice of ½ orange

3 tablespoons avocado oil

2 tablespoons white wine vinegar

2 tablespoons Almond Butter (page 150)

1 tablespoon agave syrup

Sea salt

Fresh ground black pepper

1. Rinse the quinoa thoroughly with water and cook according to the package instructions.

2. Meanwhile, cut the broccoli into florets. Bring a pot of salted water to a boil and blanch the broccoli for 3 minutes, or until bright green and crisp-tender.

3. To make the dressing, mix the orange juice, oil, vinegar, almond butter, and agave syrup in a small bowl. Season with salt and pepper.

4. Mix the spinach and quinoa in a medium bowl, then divide between two bowls. Divide the chickpeas and broccoli between the two bowls. Pour on the dressing, top with the almonds, and serve.

Health Tip

Quinoa is a pseudograin from South America, meaning "mother of all grains." It is by nature gluten-free and is an excellent source of plant protein. It contains eight different essential amino acids as well as manganese, iron, folic acid, zinc, and magnesium. Furthermore, quinoa is an important source of fiber, which we all need to retain healthy blood-fat levels and stable blood sugar levels. Quinoa provides long-lasting energy and is the perfect way to avoid hunger pangs and drowsiness.

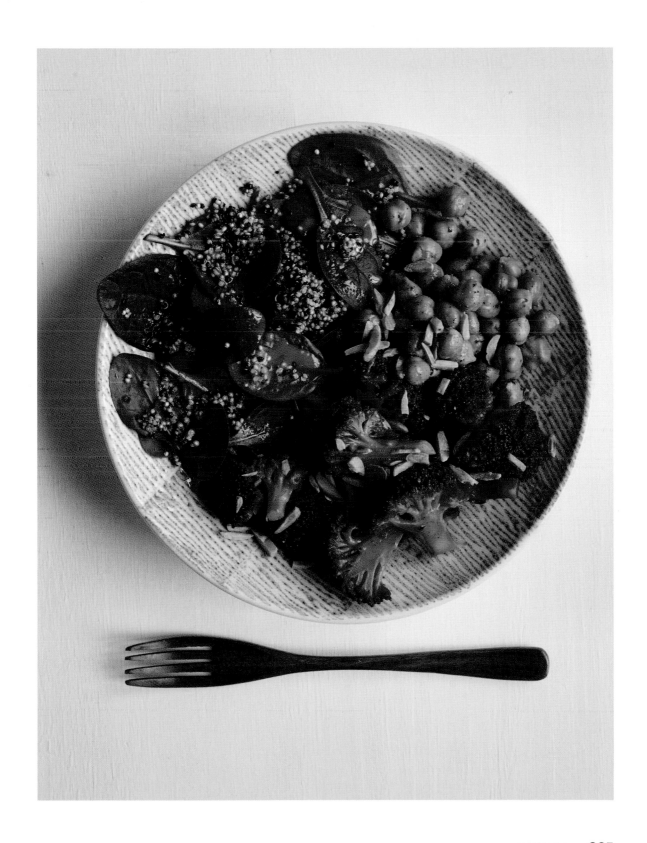

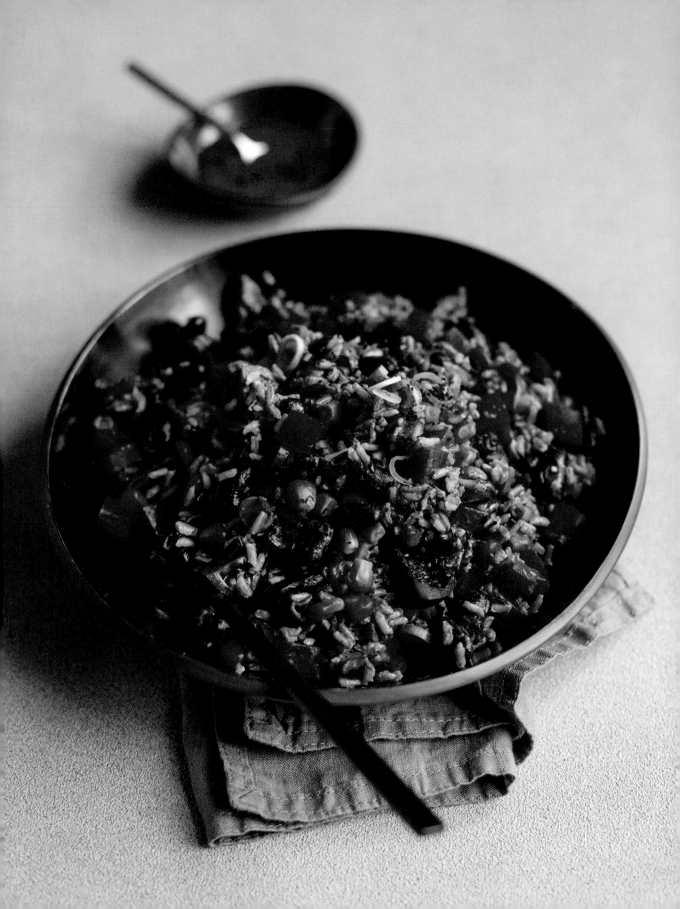

"Chili Sin Carne" Rice Salad

SERVES 2
PREP TIME: 60 minutes
PER SERVING: 560 calories, 14 g protein, 29 g fat, 61 g carbohydrates

---

⅓ cup (75 g) brown rice

1 yellow bell pepper

2 scallions

5 cherry tomatoes

¾ cup (200 g) drained, rinsed canned kidney beans

⅔ cup (100 g) drained, rinsed canned sweet corn

Sea salt

Fresh ground black pepper

DRESSING

¼ cup (60 ml) olive oil

2 tablespoons vegan sour cream

1 tablespoon tomato paste

1 teaspoon paprika

1 garlic clove

Red pepper flakes, optional

---

1. Cook the rice according to the package instructions, then set aside and let cool.

2. Meanwhile, dice the bell pepper, thinly slice the scallions, and quarter the cherry tomatoes, then transfer to a medium bowl with the beans and corn.

3. To make the dressing, mix the oil, sour cream, tomato paste, and paprika in a small bowl until creamy. Peel and press the garlic, then add it to the dressing. Season with red pepper flakes, if using.

4. Add the cooled rice to the salad, toss with the dressing, then season with salt and pepper.

Health Tip

Weighing in at 24 grams protein per 100 grams, kidney beans are one of the best sources of plant protein. If you don't tolerate legumes very well, try combining them with spices such as cumin, caraway, fennel seeds, or aniseed. Chewing them extensively before swallowing makes them much more digestible.

Creamy Yellow Lentils (*Toor dal*)

SERVES 2
PREP TIME: 30 minutes
PER SERVING: 765 calories, 44 g protein, 24 g fat, 88 g carbohydrates

---

1½ cups (300 g) yellow lentils (yellow split peas, or toor dal)

2 tomatoes

1 carrot

½ leek

1 red onion

2 tablespoons chopped parsley

DRESSING

¼ cup (60 ml) olive oil

3 tablespoons apple cider vinegar

1 teaspoon Italian seasoning

Red pepper flakes, optional

1 garlic clove

Sea salt

Fresh ground black pepper

---

1. Rinse and drain the lentils, then cook according to the package instructions.

2. Meanwhile, dice the tomatoes and carrot. Wash and thinly slice the leek. Peel and finely chop the onion. Transfer to a medium bowl.

3. Drain the cooked lentils, then add them to the bowl with the vegetables.

4. To make the dressing, combine the oil, vinegar, Italian seasoning, and red pepper flakes, if using, in a small bowl. Peel and press the garlic and add it to the dressing, then season with salt and pepper.

5. Pour the dressing over the salad and toss to combine. Divide between bowls, top with the parsley, and serve.

Health Tip

Yellow lentils, or rather, yellow split peas, are generally already hulled and are thus more easily digested than other types of legumes, making them ideal for anyone who may have previously avoided lentils because of worries about flatulence. They become creamy when cooked and have a very mild taste. Like all legumes, they are high in protein.

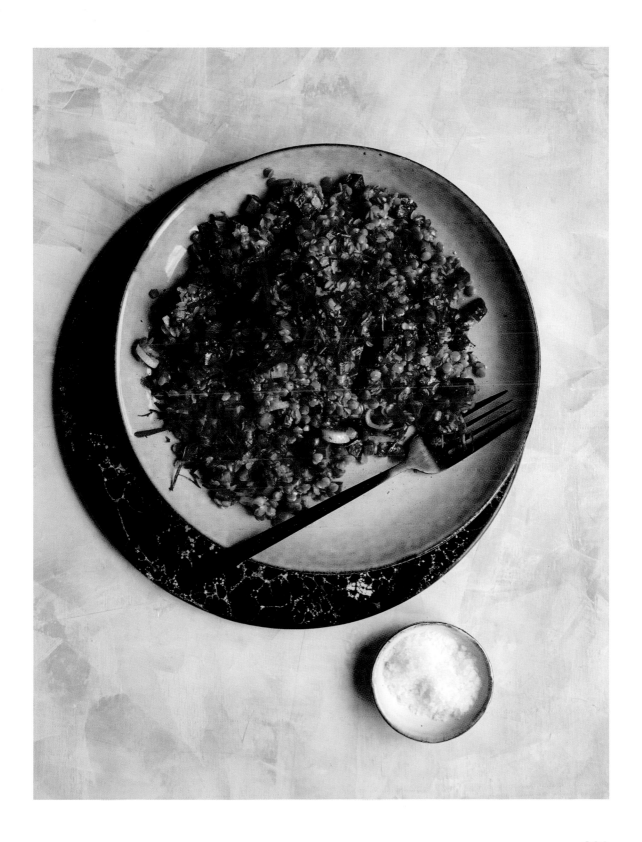

Tofu Palak "Paneer"

SERVES 2
PREP TIME: 30 minutes
PER SERVING: 515 calories, 32 g protein,
36 g fat, 20 g carbohydrates

---

14 ounces (400 g) firm tofu
1 pound (450 g) spinach
2 garlic cloves
1-inch (2.5 cm) piece ginger
2 jalapeños
1 red onion
2 tomatoes
¼ cup (60 ml) coconut oil
1 tablespoon ground cumin
2 teaspoons ground cinnamon
1 teaspoon ground cardamom
1 teaspoon garam masala
Sea salt
Fresh ground black pepper

---

1. Drain the tofu, then sandwich between several layers of kitchen towels to remove excess liquid.

2. Bring a pot of salted water to a boil and blanch the spinach until just wilted, about 1 minute. Drain and transfer immediately to a bowl of ice water to stop the cooking. Drain and transfer to a blender.

3. Peel and coarsely chop the garlic and ginger. Stem and seed the jalapeños. Add to the blender and blend until a smooth paste forms.

4. Peel and finely chop the onion. Dice the tomatoes and tofu.

5. Heat the oil in a medium pot over medium heat and add the cumin, cinnamon, cardamom, and garam masala. Cook until fragrant, about 2 minutes. Add the onion and tomatoes and cook for another 5 minutes.

6. Stir in the spinach paste and tofu along with 1 cup (240 ml) water and simmer over low heat for 5 minutes.

7. Season with salt and pepper, divide between bowls, and serve, alone or with brown basmati rice.

Health Tip
Spinach is a fast-growing plant that absorbs many nutrients from the ground. For your body to better incorporate these nutrients, combine spinach with other foods rich in vitamin C, such as tomatoes or broccoli.

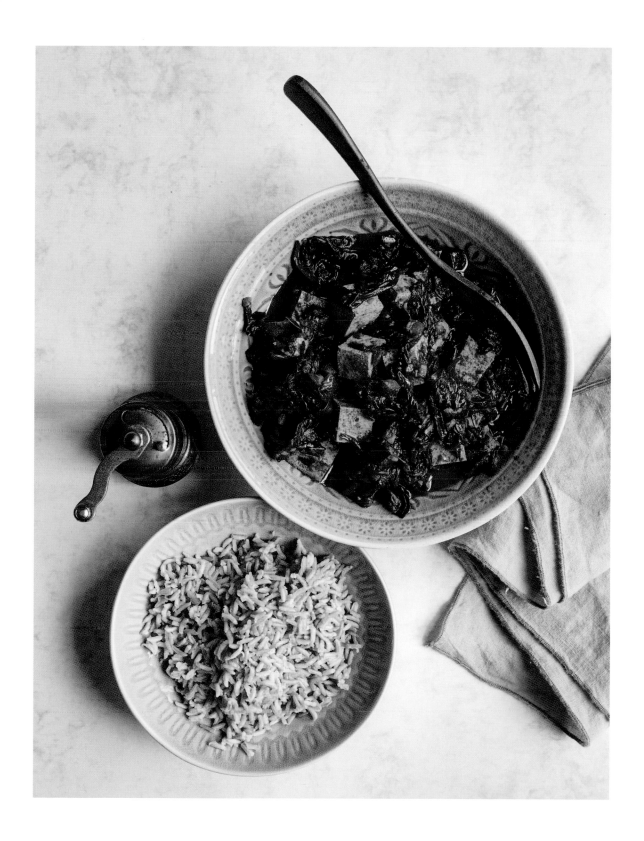

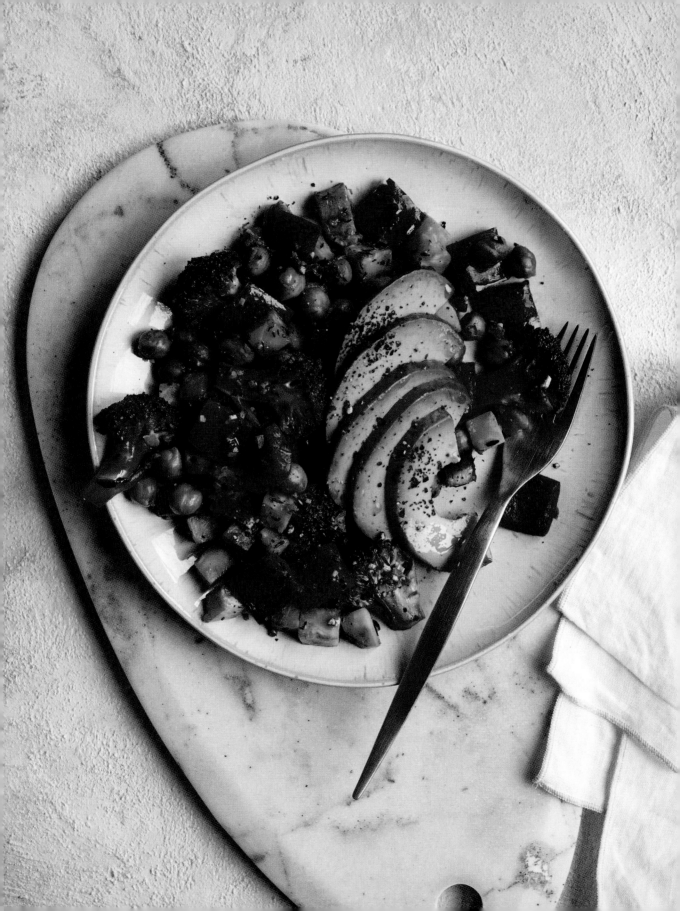

Celery Root Sauté

SERVES 2
PREP TIME: 30 minutes
PER SERVING: 480 calories, 15 g protein,
35 g fat, 25 g carbohydrates

---

14 ounces (400 g) celery root
2 yellow bell peppers
10½ ounces (300 g) broccoli
1 scallion
2 garlic cloves
2 tablespoons canola oil
1 cup (200 g) drained, rinsed canned
   chickpeas
1 tablespoon dried thyme
Sea salt
Fresh ground black pepper
Red pepper flakes, optional
1 avocado

---

1. Peel and dice the celery root, dice the bell peppers, and cut the broccoli into florets. Finely chop the scallion. Peel and finely chop the garlic.

2. Heat the oil in a medium skillet over medium heat, add the garlic and scallion, and cook for 3 minutes. Add the celery root, broccoli, and bell peppers, and cook for another 5 minutes. Add the chickpeas and cook for another 2 minutes.

3. Season with the thyme, salt, and pepper. Add ⅔ cup (160 ml) water and simmer for 10 minutes. Season with red pepper flakes, if using, then remove from the heat.

4. Divide between two bowls. Halve, pit, peel, and slice the avocado, then place on top of the stir-fry and serve.

> ### Health Tip
> Celery, from the root to the stalk, is a true health miracle. It detoxes, inhibits inflammation, lowers blood pressure, and regulates digestion. And it delivers important B vitamins, calcium, and potassium, all while also keeping us hydrated.

Pea Soup

SERVES 2
PREP TIME: 50 minutes
PER SERVING: 280 calories, 11 g protein,
15 g fat, 19 g carbohydrates

---

1 onion

1 large carrot

1 celery rib

2 tablespoons coconut oil

1⅓ cups (200 g) green peas, fresh or
frozen

2 to 3 tablespoons Vegetable Broth Paste
(page 174)

Sea salt

Fresh ground black pepper

2 tablespoons pumpkin seeds

---

1. Peel and dice the onion. Dice the carrot and celery.

2. Heat the oil in a medium pot and cook the onion, carrot, and celery for 3 minutes.

3. Add the broth paste and 4 cups (1 L) water and bring to a boil. Lower the heat, cover, and simmer for 30 minutes. Add the peas and cook for 10 minutes more.

4. Season with salt and pepper. Divide between two bowls and top with the pumpkin seeds. Serve alone or with Pumpkin Seed and Chia Bread (page 158).

Health Tip

Peas may be tiny, but they are an unbelievably healthy food. They help to lower cholesterol and lipid levels in the blood, and they have a positive effect on digestion. The fiber in peas absorbs bile in the intestine. And, like other legumes, peas have one of the highest levels of protein of all plant-based foods.

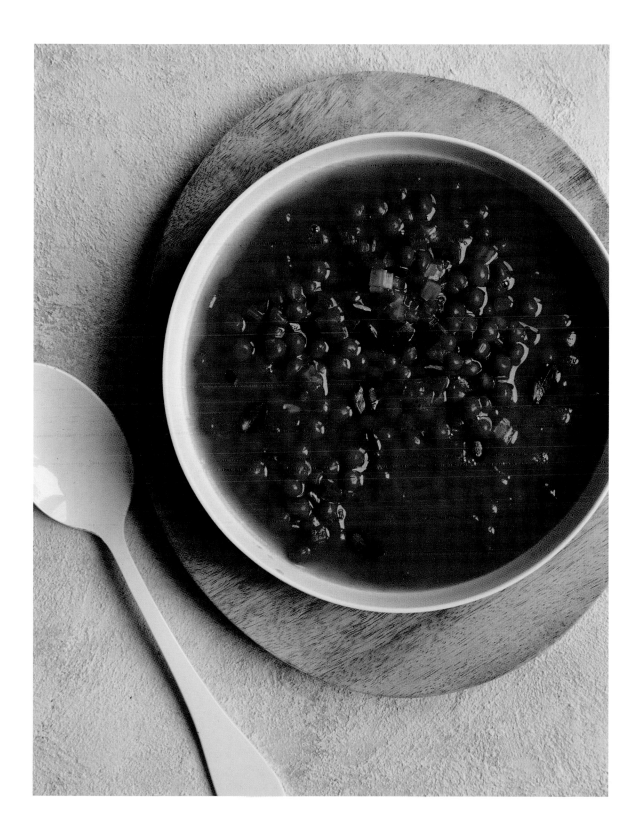

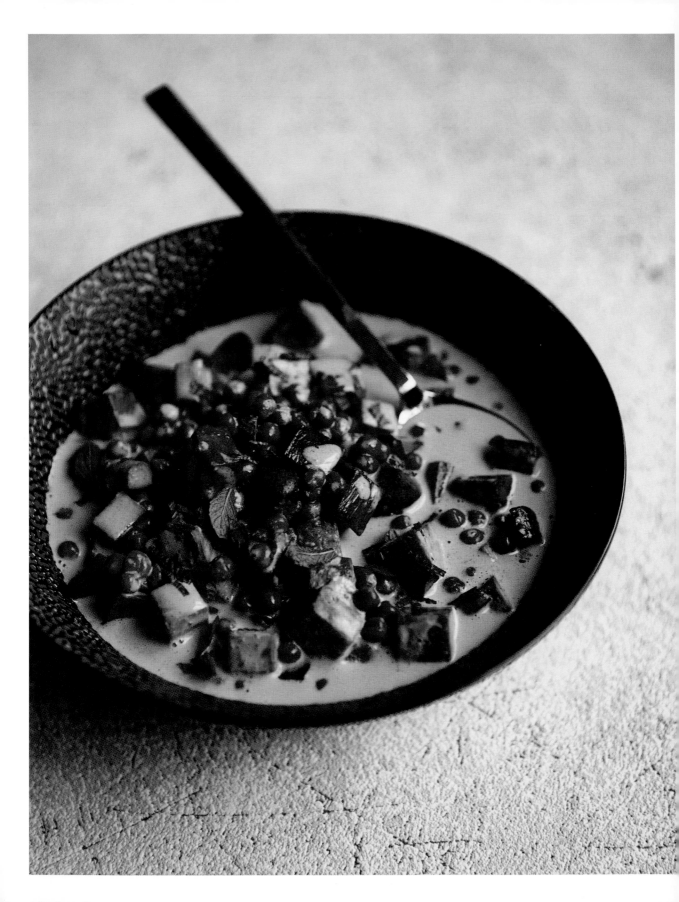

Sweet Potato and Green Pea Curry

SERVES 2
PREP TIME: 40 minutes
PER SERVING: 670 calories, 14 g protein, 41 g fat, 61 g carbohydrates

1 carrot
1 large sweet potato
1 tablespoon coconut oil
2 teaspoons curry powder
1 teaspoon ground fennel seeds
½ teaspoon ground anise seeds
½ teaspoon ground caraway seeds
⅔ cup (100 g) green peas, fresh or frozen
1 cup (240 ml) coconut milk
1 tablespoon Almond Butter (page 150)
1 teaspoon sea salt
2 tablespoons chopped mint

1. Dice the carrot and sweet potato into bite-size cubes.

2. Heat the oil in a large pot over medium heat. Add the curry powder, fennel, anise, and caraway and cook until fragrant, stirring constantly, for about 1 minute. Add the carrot, sweet potatoes, and peas and cook for 5 minutes, stirring occasionally.

3. Add the coconut milk, almond butter, and 1 cup (240 ml) water. Simmer for 15 minutes, then stir in the salt.

4. Remove from the heat and let the curry rest and thicken in the pot for about 10 minutes.

5. Divide between two bowls, sprinkle with the mint, and serve alone or with wild rice.

Health Tip

Curry powder is not a stand-alone spice but rather a mixture of some thirty healthy spices. The most common ingredients are turmeric, coriander, cumin, fenugreek, ginger, nutmeg, cayenne pepper, cardamom, fennel, cinnamon, and cloves. Curry powder and curry paste achieve their full flavor when mixed with fats.

Root Vegetable Curry

SERVES 2
PREP TIME: 45 minutes
PER SERVING: 500 calories, 11 g protein, 35 g fat, 32 g carbohydrates

---

1 large rutabaga
1 parsnip
1 beet
1 red onion
1 garlic clove
1-inch (2.5 cm) piece ginger
½ red chile, seeded for less heat
1 tablespoon Almond Butter (page 150)
2 tablespoons sesame oil
2 tablespoons soy sauce
1 cup (140 g) peeled, diced potatoes
¾ cup (180 ml) coconut milk

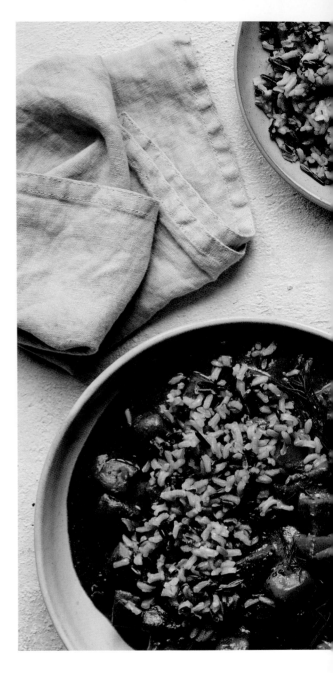

1. Peel and dice the rutabaga, parsnip, and beet.

2. Peel and coarsely chop the onion, garlic, and ginger and transfer to a food processor. Add the chile, almond butter, sesame oil, soy sauce, and ¼ cup (60 ml) water and blend until a creamy paste forms.

3. Transfer the paste to a medium skillet over medium-high heat and cook for about 5 minutes. Add the potato, rutabaga, parsnip, and beet and cook for another 5 minutes, stirring occasionally.

4. Deglaze with the coconut milk, then add ½ cup (120 ml) water and simmer over low heat for 20 minutes, until thickened. Remove from the heat, divide between bowls, and serve plain or over brown basmati and wild rice.

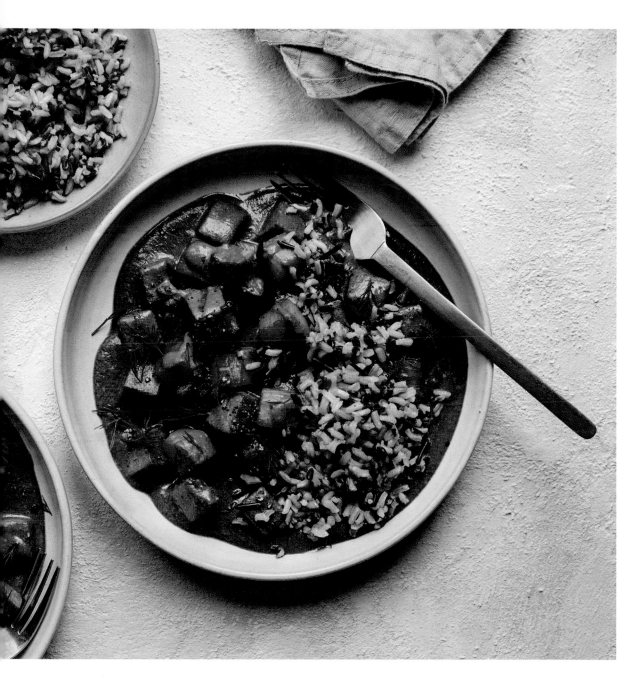

Health Tip

The pigment from red beets, betaine, has a strong antioxidant effect and prevents cell damage. Betaine also acts against inflammatory processes and stimulates the liver cells, removing toxins from the body and supporting the body's own immune system. Red beets also prevent deposits from affixing to the lining of blood vessels.

Turmeric Curry with Rice Noodles

SERVES 2
PREP TIME: 45 minutes
PER SERVING: 810 calories, 29 g protein, 58 g fat, 69 g carbohydrates

TURMERIC PASTE
2 fresh turmeric roots, or 2 tablespoons ground turmeric
1 onion
1-inch (2.5 cm) piece ginger
1 garlic clove
1 large tomato

CURRY
3½ ounces (100 g) green beans
1 handful cremini mushrooms
1 scallion
7 ounces (200 g) smoked tofu
½ bunch cilantro
3 tablespoons coconut oil
1 cup (240 ml) coconut milk
2 tablespoons sesame oil
1 tablespoon agave syrup
1 tablespoon soy sauce
3½ ounces (100 g) rice noodles
1 handful bean sprouts

1. To prepare the turmeric paste, peel and dice the turmeric roots, onion, garlic, and ginger. Dice the tomato. Transfer to a food processor and blend until smooth.

2. To make the curry, halve the green beans, quarter the mushrooms, and thinly slice the scallion. Dice the tofu and finely chop the cilantro.

3. Heat 1 tablespoon of the oil in a medium skillet over medium-high heat and fry the tofu until crisp, about 7 to 10 minutes, stirring regularly. Remove from the heat and set aside.

4. Heat the remaining 2 tablespoons oil in a large pot over medium heat, add the turmeric paste, and cook for 2 minutes. Add the green beans and mushrooms and cook for another 2 minutes.

4. Deglaze with the coconut milk and simmer over low heat for 10 minutes. Stir in the sesame oil, agave syrup, and soy sauce and remove from the heat.

5. While the curry simmers, cook the noodles according to the package instructions.

6. Divide the noodles and curry between two bowls, top with the scallion, tofu, sprouts, and cilantro, and serve.

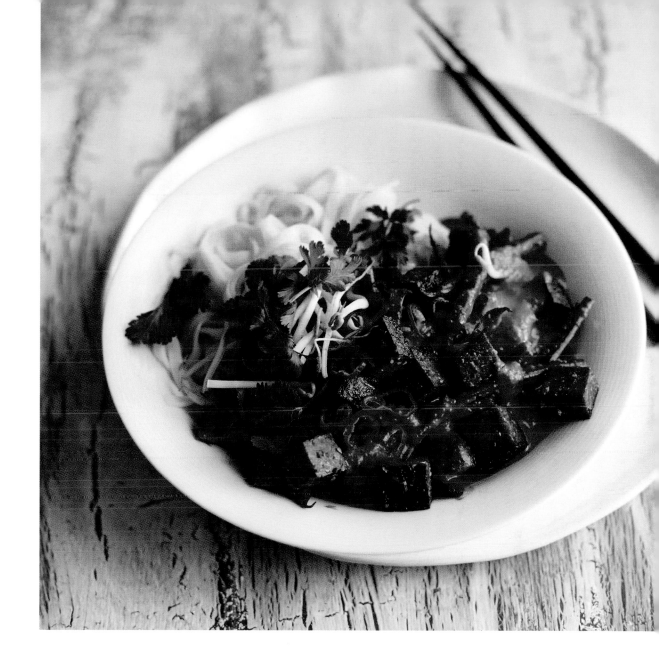

Health Tip

Turmeric eases intestinal symptoms such as bloating, heartburn, diarrhea, constipation, flatulence, and cramps. It has an anti-inflammatory effect, which can help with skin problems and acne. The main active ingredient in turmeric is curcumin, which gives it its intense bright color. Since it can also discolor your hands, you may want to use gloves when preparing the fresh root.

Indian-Spiced Lentils (*Moong dal*)

SERVES 2
PREP TIME: 45 minutes
PER SERVING: 890 calories, 41 g protein, 66 g fat, 64 g carbohydrates

---

7 ounces (200 g) firm tofu
1 garlic clove
1-inch (2.5 cm) piece ginger
½ jalapeño, seeded for less heat
14 ounces (400 g) fresh spinach
3 tablespoons peanut oil
1 teaspoon ground cumin
3 tablespoons coconut oil
1 red onion
2 tomatoes
1 teaspoon ground cardamom
1 teaspoon ground cinnamon
1 teaspoon garam masala
1 cup (240 ml) coconut milk
¾ cup (150 g) petite yellow lentils
   (*moong dal*)

---

1. Drain the tofu, then sandwich between several layers of kitchen towels to remove excess liquid. Peel and coarsely chop the garlic and ginger.

2. Transfer the ginger, garlic, jalapeño, and half of the spinach to a blender along with the peanut oil and blend until smooth.

3. Dice the tofu, transfer to a medium bowl with the cumin, and mix well.

4. Heat 1 tablespoon of the coconut oil in a medium skillet over medium-high heat and fry the tofu until crispy, about 7 to 10 minutes. Remove from the heat and set aside.

5. Peel and finely chop the onion and dice the tomatoes.

6. Add the remaining 2 tablespoons coconut oil to a pot over medium-high heat, then add the spinach paste. Add the onion, tomatoes, cardamom, cinnamon, and garam masala and cook for 2 minutes.

7. Deglaze with the coconut milk and 1 cup (240 ml) water. Add the lentils and stir thoroughly. Bring to a boil, then turn the heat to low, cover, and simmer for 15 minutes.

8. Stir in the remaining spinach, then remove from the heat and let rest and thicken for 10 minutes. Serve topped with the tofu.

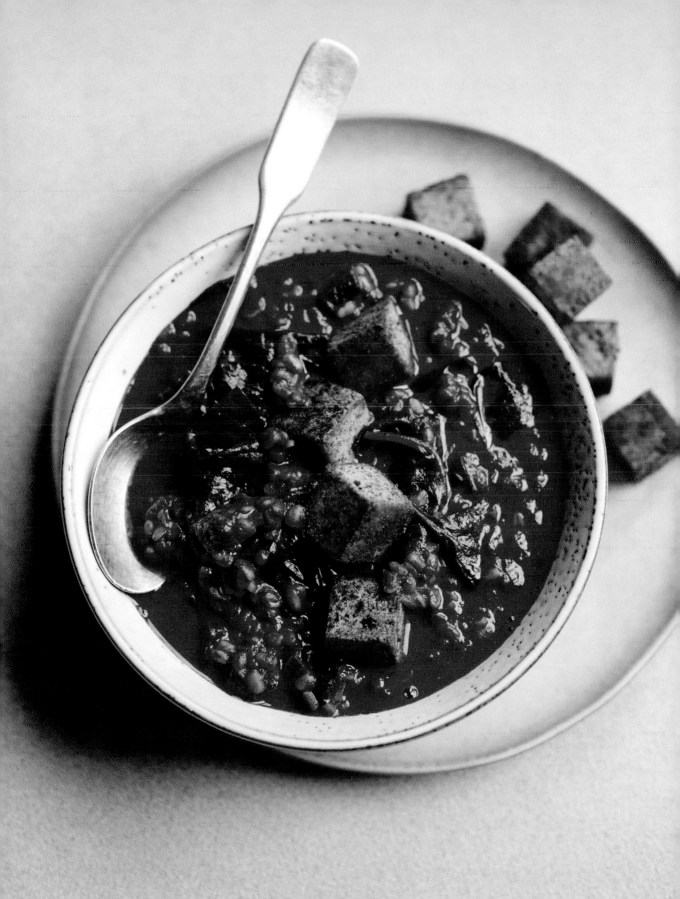

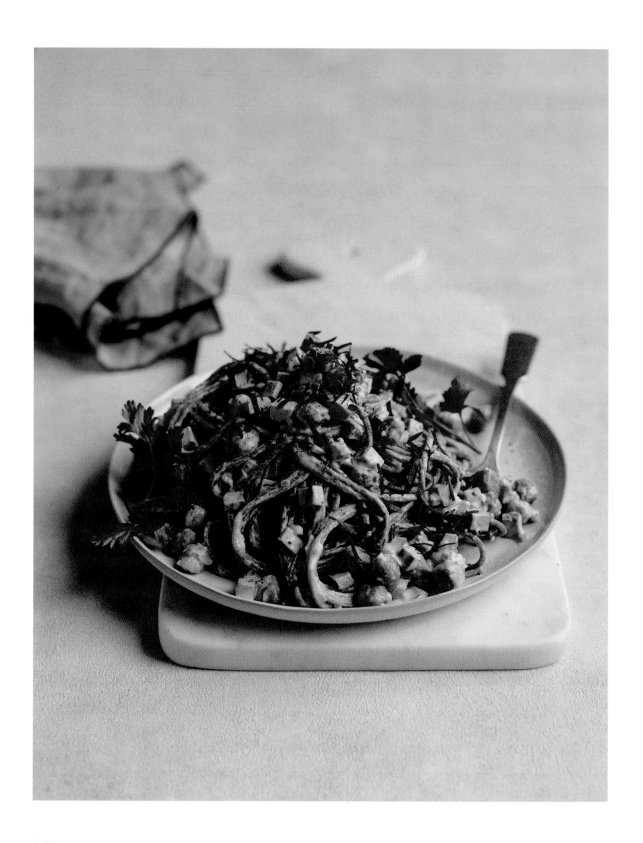

Chickpea Carbonara

SERVES 2
PREP TIME: 25 minutes
PER SERVING: 1,630 calories, 56 g protein, 86 g fat, 216 g carbohydrates

---

1 pound (450 g) spelt spaghetti

1 onion

2 garlic cloves

7 ounces (200 g) smoked tofu

1 bunch parsley

1 tablespoon canola oil

1¼ cups (250 g) drained, rinsed canned chickpeas

1¼ cup (280 g) vegan sour cream

Sea salt

Fresh ground black pepper

1 teaspoon ground nutmeg

---

1. Cook the spaghetti according to the package instructions. Drain and set aside.

2. While the pasta cooks, peel and chop the onion and garlic, and dice the tofu. Finely chop the parsley.

3. Heat the oil in a large skillet and fry the onion, garlic, and tofu for 5 minutes. Add the chickpeas and cook for another 3 minutes.

4. Add the sour cream and 1 cup (240 ml) water and let the mixture simmer for 2 more minutes, stirring regularly.

5. Add the spaghetti and mix well. Season with salt, pepper, and the nutmeg. Divide between two dishes, sprinkle with the parsley, and serve.

Health Tip

We love parsley! It is an active diuretic, supports digestion, and inhibits inflammation. Fun fact: If you chew on a few leaves after eating, you can get rid of garlic breath.

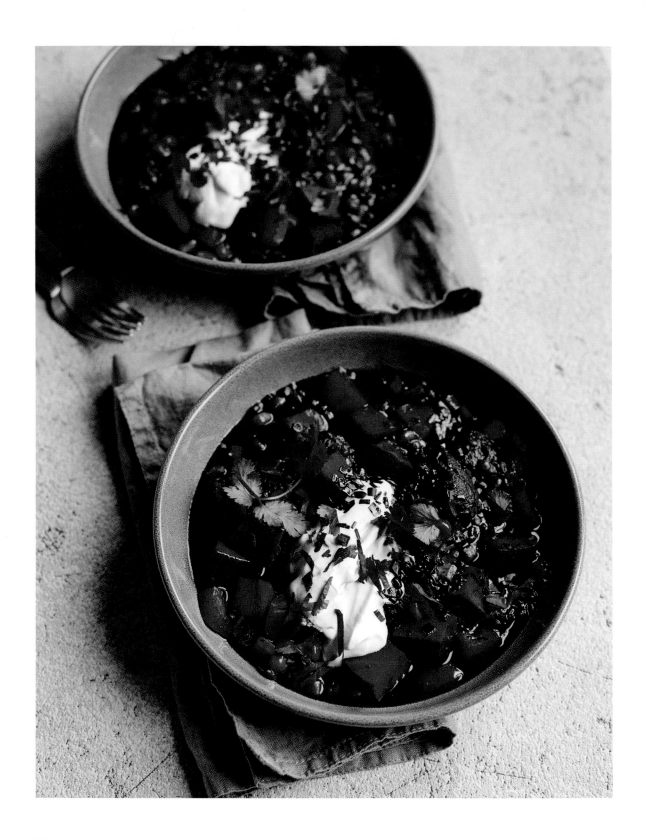

Lentil-Chocolate Chili

SERVES 2
PREP TIME: 50 minutes
PER SERVING: 550 calories, 22 g protein, 21 g fat, 66 g carbohydrates

---

1 red onion
1 garlic clove
½ yellow bell pepper
1 tablespoon coconut oil
1 teaspoon ground cumin
1 teaspoon paprika
1 teaspoon dried thyme
1 teaspoon chili paste
½ cup (100 g) brown lentils
1½ cups (200 g) cubed red kuri or butternut squash
⅔ cup (100 g) drained, rinsed canned sweet corn
2 tablespoons raw cacao powder
¾ cup (200 g) canned whole peeled tomatoes
2 teaspoons Vegetable Broth Paste (page 174)
½ bunch cilantro
2 teaspoons vegan sour cream
2 tablespoons grated vegan dark chocolate (80 percent cocoa)

---

1. Peel and finely dice the onion and garlic. Dice the bell pepper.

2. Heat the oil in a small pot over medium heat, add the onion and garlic, and cook for 3 minutes, stirring constantly, until the onion is translucent.

3. Add the cumin, paprika, thyme, and chili paste and cook for another 5 minutes, stirring occasionally.

4. Rinse and drain the lentils, then add them to the pot and cook for 1 minute, stirring constantly.

5. Add the squash, bell pepper, corn, and cacao and mix well. Add the tomatoes, 1 cup (240 ml) water, and the broth paste and bring the mixture to a boil. Turn the heat to low, cover, and simmer over low heat for 25 minutes, stirring occasionally.

6. Meanwhile, finely chop the cilantro.

7. Remove the chili from the heat and divide between two bowls. Top with the sour cream, cilantro, and chocolate and serve.

Health Tip
Raw cacao has an extremely high magnesium content. It protects the cells with antioxidants and provides us with lots of calcium. It can also lower blood pressure, help digestion, and increase concentration. But above all, it's a happy food! Chocolate supports the body in the production of endorphins (happiness hormones).

Red Lentils with Spinach

SERVES 2
PREP TIME: 40 minutes
PER SERVING: 430 calories, 18 g protein,
21 g fat, 42 g carbohydrates

---

1 red onion
1 garlic clove
1-inch (2.5 cm) piece ginger
2 tablespoons coconut oil
1 teaspoon curry powder
½ teaspoon red pepper flakes
1 tart apple
½ cup (100 g) red lentils
1 cup (200 g) canned diced tomatoes
Scant ½ cup (100 ml) coconut milk
3 handfuls spinach
Sea salt
Fresh ground black pepper

---

1. Peel and finely dice the onion, garlic, and ginger.

2. Heat the oil in a large pot over medium-high heat and sauté the onion, garlic, and ginger for 3 minutes until softened, stirring occasionally. Add the curry powder and red pepper flakes and mix well. Cook for an additional 2 minutes.

3. Quarter, core and finely dice the apple. Rinse and drain the lentils. Add to the pot.

4. Stir in the tomatoes, coconut milk, and a scant 1 cup (200 ml) water and bring the mixture to a boil. Turn the heat to low, cover, and simmer for 20 minutes.

5. Remove from the heat and let cool, then add the spinach and season with salt and pepper. Divide between bowls and serve.

Health Tip

Red lentils contain many valuable nutrients and are very filling. They're rich in iron, which is critical for our circulatory system and the health of our muscles and liver. These mild-tasting legumes are home to many bioactive substances, such as saponins, flavonoids, and polyphenols, which can lower the cholesterol level in the blood. They're also said to lower the risk of several cancers.

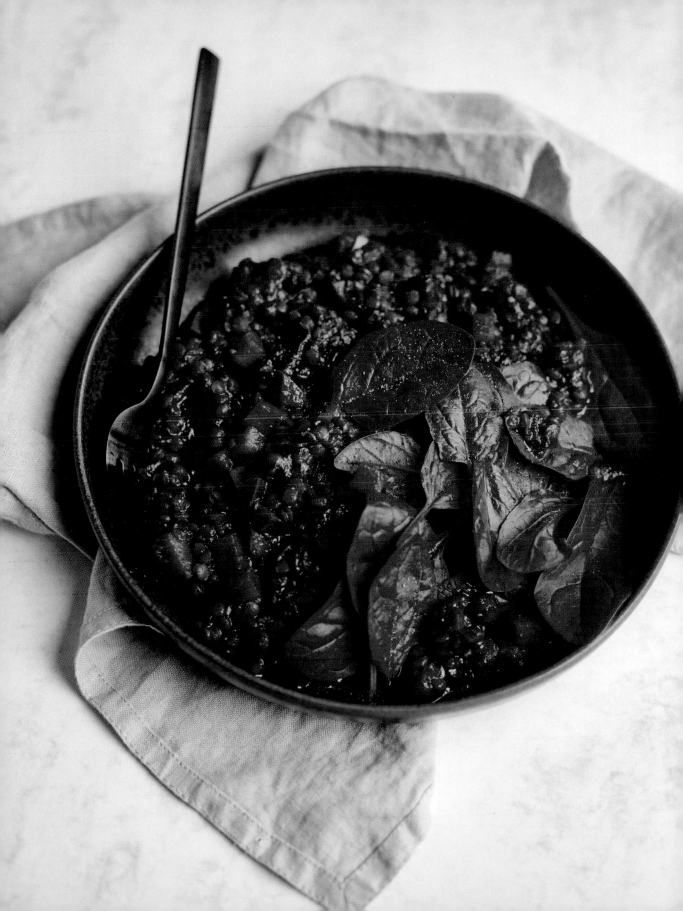

Dessert

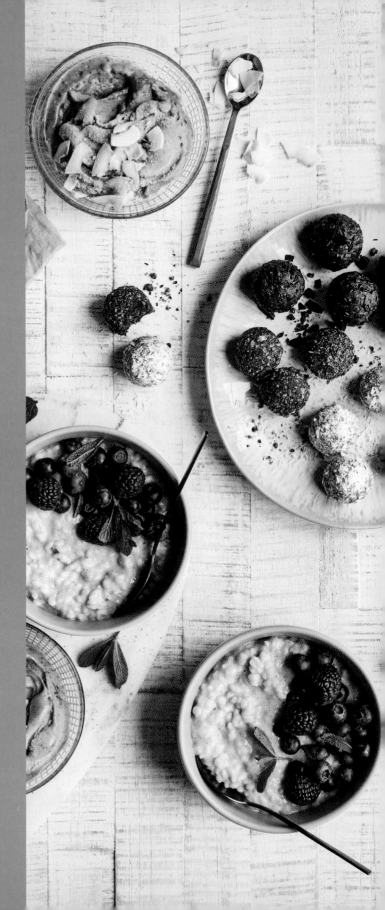

Sweet Potato and Chocolate Pudding

SERVES 2
PREP TIME: 30 minutes
PER SERVING: 360 calories, 9 g protein, 19 g fat, 38 g carbohydrates

½ sweet potato
1 tablespoon chia seeds
1 tablespoon Almond Butter (page 150)
4 Medjool dates, pitted
3 tablespoons raw cacao powder
⅓ cup (75 ml) Almond Milk (page 145)
Shredded coconut
Pomegranate seeds

1. Fill a small pot with water and boil the sweet potato for 20 minutes.

2. Transfer the sweet potato to a blender along with the chia seeds, almond butter, dates, cacao powder, and almond milk and blend until smooth.

3. Divide the pudding between two bowls, top with the coconut and pomegranate seeds, and serve.

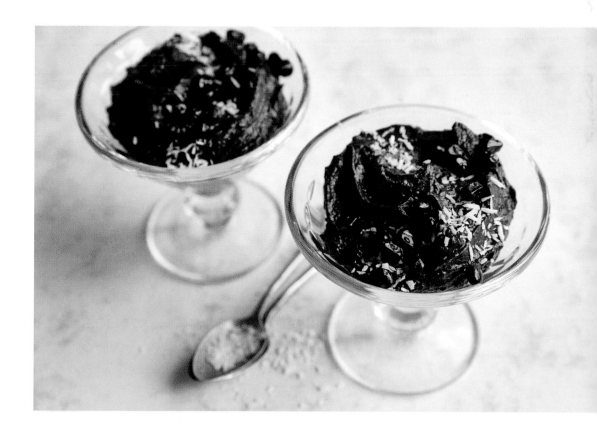

Coconut Rice Pudding

SERVES 2
PREP TIME: 30 minutes
PER SERVING: 430 calories, 7 g protein, 22 g fat, 49 g carbohydrates

Scant 1 cup (200 ml) Cashew Milk (page 145)
Scant 1 cup (200 ml) coconut milk
⅓ cup (60 g) short-grain white rice
2 tablespoons coconut sugar
2 teaspoons ground cinnamon
Pinch of ground cardamom
Pinch of sea salt
Fresh berries
Mint leaves

1. Combine the cashew milk and coconut milk in a medium pot and bring to a boil. Add the rice, sugar, cinnamon, cardamom, and salt, then turn the heat to low and cook according to the rice package instructions, stirring occasionally.

2. Divide the rice between two small bowls. Top with the berries and mint and serve.

> ### Health Tip
> Coconut milk comes from the flesh of coconuts, not from the liquid, which is called coconut water. The flesh, once removed, is ground up, pressed, and strained. Coconut milk is very nutritious. It has a high fat percentage (20 percent), but these are healthy fats—medium-chain triglycerides, or MCTs, which are easily digested and turned into energy. Coconut milk is a good alternative to dairy milk and cream in desserts. It is also excellent in soups, stews, and curries.

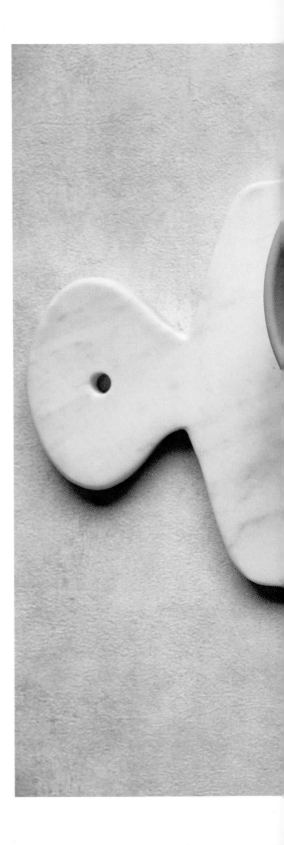

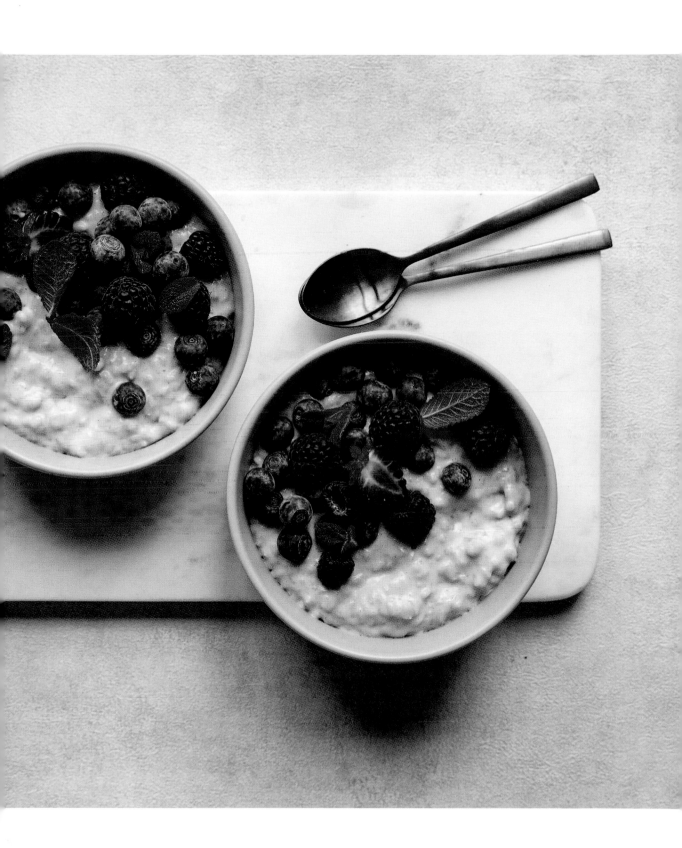

Oatmeal Cookies

MAKES 15 COOKIES
PREP TIME: 20 minutes
BAKING TIME: 15 minutes
PER COOKIE: 85 calories, 3 g protein,
4 g fat, 10 g carbohydrates

1⅔ cups (150 g) rolled oats
½ cup (50 g) coconut sugar
½ teaspoon baking powder
1 teaspoon Bourbon vanilla extract
½ teaspoon almond extract
⅓ cup (80 g) Almond Butter (page 150)
⅓ cup (90 ml) Almond Milk (page 145)
2 tablespoons coconut nectar or maple
   syrup

1. Preheat the oven to 350°F (180°C). Line a baking sheet with parchment paper.

2. Pour half of the oats into a food processor and grind finely, then transfer to a medium bowl with the remaining oats, sugar, baking powder, vanilla, and almond extract.

3. Carefully heat the almond butter in a small pot over medium-low heat. Add the almond milk and coconut nectar and stir well.

4. Pour the wet ingredients into the bowl and mix until a sticky dough forms.

5. Transfer tablespoon-size balls of dough, one at a time, onto the baking sheet, about 2 inches apart. With the back of a wet spoon, flatten the balls into nice round cookies.

6. Bake for 10 minutes, or until golden brown. Remove from the oven, transfer to a cooling rack, and enjoy.

Health Tip

Bourbon vanilla comes from Madagascar and Réunion Island (formerly known as Bourbon Island) and is produced from the pod of a type of orchid. Freshly harvested, the vanilla pods have virtually no taste to them, since the flavor develops only through heat and fermentation. Naturally grown vanilla is antiseptic and anti-inflammatory and can be a mood enhancer. If you buy whole vanilla pods, choose long and elastic ones, since dry and hardened pods may have already lost their flavor.

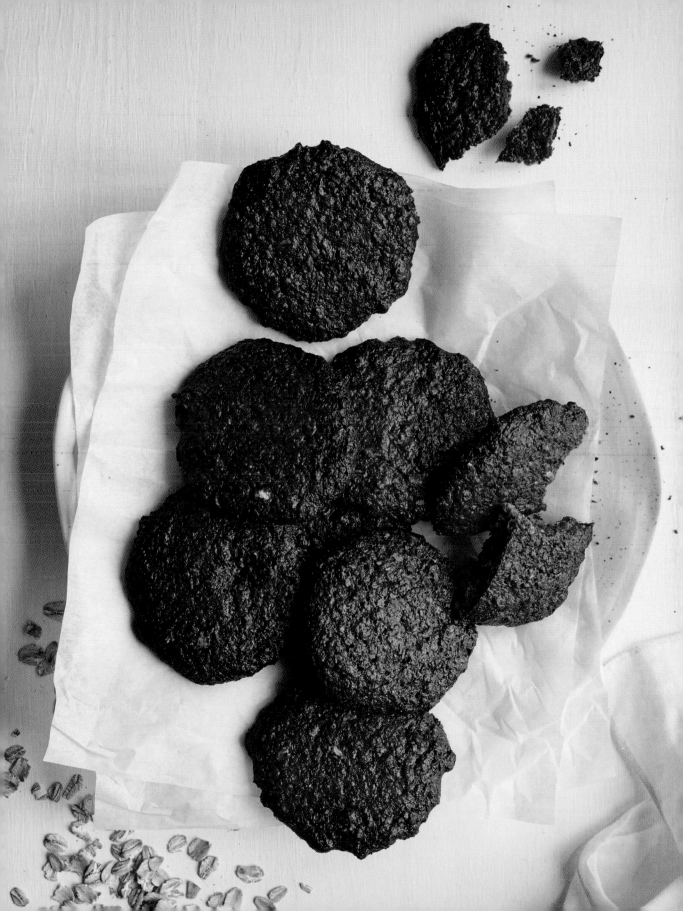

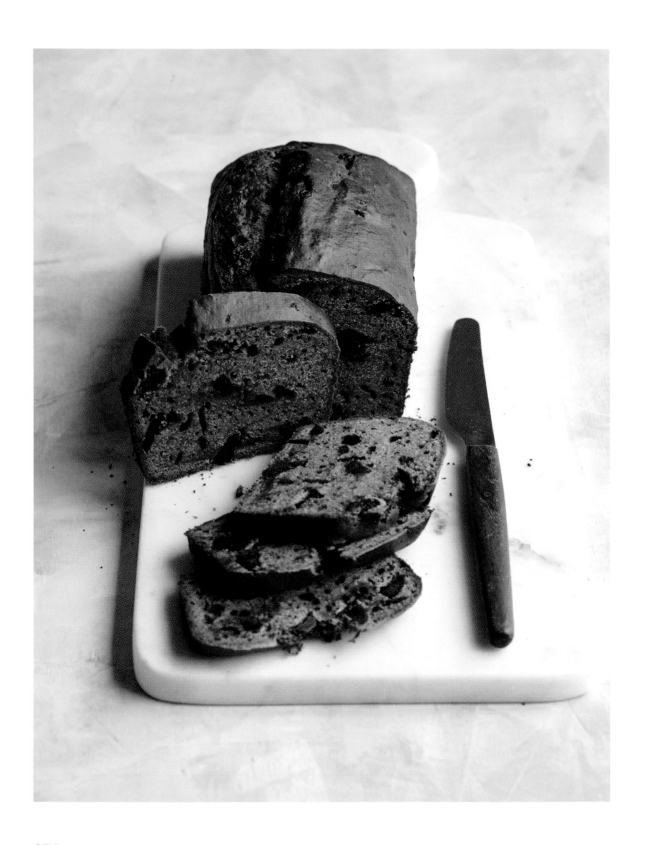

Banana Bread

MAKES ONE 9 × 5-INCH (23 × 13 CM) LOAF
PREP TIME: 15 minutes
BAKING TIME: 60 minutes
PER SERVING (½-INCH/1 CM SLICE): 255 calories, 6 g protein, 10 g fat, 35 g carbohydrates

---

2 tablespoons coconut oil, plus extra for greasing

2½ cups (300 g) spelt flour

½ cup (50 g) coconut sugar

1 tablespoon baking powder

2 teaspoons ground cinnamon

2 ounces (60 g) vegan dark chocolate (at least 80 percent cocoa)

3 ripe bananas

Scant ½ cup (100 ml) Almond Milk (page 145)

3 tablespoons Almond Butter (page 150)

1 tablespoon apple cider vinegar

Pinch of sea salt

---

1. Preheat the oven to 350°F (180°C). Brush a 9 x 5-inch (23 x 13 cm) loaf pan with oil.

2. Mix the flour, sugar, baking powder, and cinnamon in a medium bowl. Chop the chocolate.

3. Peel the bananas and place in a blender with the 2 tablespoons oil, the almond milk, almond butter, vinegar, and salt. Blend until smooth.

4. Transfer to the bowl with the dry ingredients and mix until a smooth batter forms.

5. Pour into the pan and smooth the surface with a wet spoon. Bake for 1 hour, or until golden brown.

6. Remove from the oven and let cool in the pan for at least 20 minutes, then transfer to a cooling rack before serving.

Health Tip

Bananas are a quick natural source of energy and are rich in potassium, magnesium, and vitamin B_6. They can also act as a mood enhancer and stress reliever, because of the amino acid tryptophan, which the body transforms into the happiness hormone serotonin. The pectin in bananas helps to bind fluid in the intestine and thus prevents digestive problems.

Aquafaba Chocolate Mousse

SERVES 2
PREP TIME: 20 minutes
COOLING TIME: 1 hour
PER SERVING: 175 calories, 4 g protein, 12 g fat, 13 g carbohydrates

---

⅔ cup (150 ml) aquafaba (liquid from a can of chickpeas)

3½ ounces (100 g) vegan dark chocolate, plus extra for serving

2 tablespoons coconut sugar

1 tablespoon raw cacao powder

½ teaspoon Bourbon vanilla extract

---

1. Mix the aquafaba with an electric mixer until stiff peaks form, about 5 minutes.

2. Melt the chocolate in a double boiler over hot water. Add the sugar, cacao powder, and vanilla and stir to combine. Remove from the heat and let cool.

3. Gradually fold the whipped aquafaba into the chocolate mixture, stirring after each addition.

4. Divide between two glasses and refrigerate for at least 1 hour (the longer, the better). Chop or shave the extra chocolate, sprinkle on top, and serve.

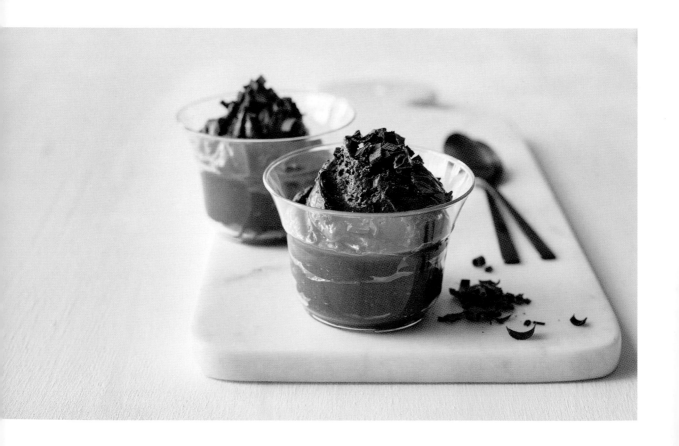

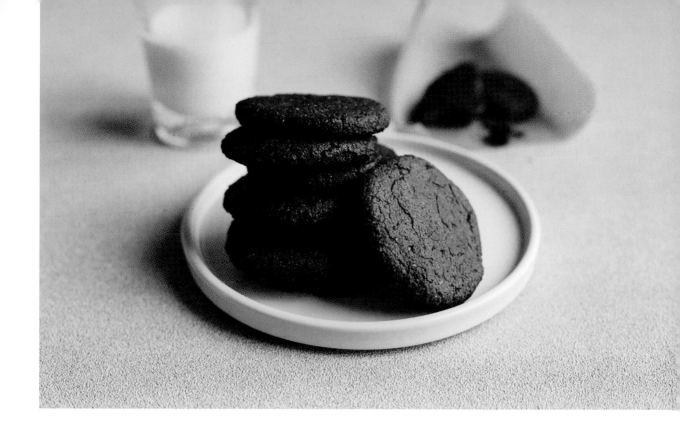

Avocado Cookies

MAKES 10 COOKIES
PREP TIME: 20 minutes
BAKING TIME: 15 minutes
PER COOKIE: 110 calories, 2 g protein,
7 g fat, 10 g carbohydrates

1 avocado
1 teaspoon lemon juice
1⅔ cups (200 g) spelt flour
¾ cup plus 1½ tablespoons (100 g)
   coconut flour
¼ cup (45 g) coconut sugar
2 tablespoons coconut oil, melted
1 tablespoon raw cacao powder
½ teaspoon baking powder
½ teaspoon Bourbon vanilla extract
Pinch of sea salt

1. Preheat the oven to 350°F (180°C). Line a baking sheet with parchment paper.

2. Halve, pit, and peel the avocado, then transfer to a medium bowl and mash with a fork. Add the lemon juice and stir to combine.

3. Add the remaining ingredients and mix until a smooth dough forms.

4. Transfer tablespoon-size balls of dough, one at a time, onto the baking sheet, about 2 inches apart. With the back of a wet spoon, flatten the balls into nice round cookies.

5. Bake for 10 minutes, or until golden brown, then remove and cool on a wire rack before serving.

Banana-Coconut Nice Cream

SERVES 2
PREP TIME: 10 minutes
PER SERVING: 390 calories, 8 g protein, 21 g fat, 42 g carbohydrates

3 frozen (very ripe) bananas, peeled before freezing
3 Medjool dates, pitted and chopped
¼ cup (60 ml) coconut milk
2 tablespoons Almond Butter (page 150)
1 teaspoon cinnamon
1 teaspoon Bourbon vanilla extract
½ teaspoon ground cardamom
Coconut chips

1. Blend the bananas, dates, coconut milk, almond butter, cinnamon, vanilla, and cardamom in a blender until creamy.

2. Divide between bowls, top with coconut chips, and serve immediately.

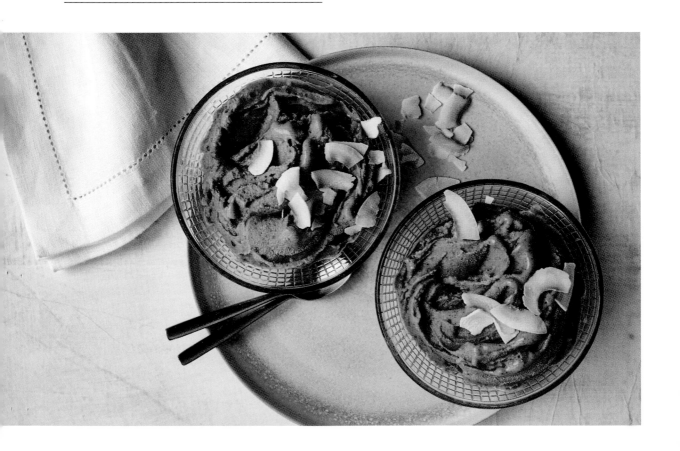

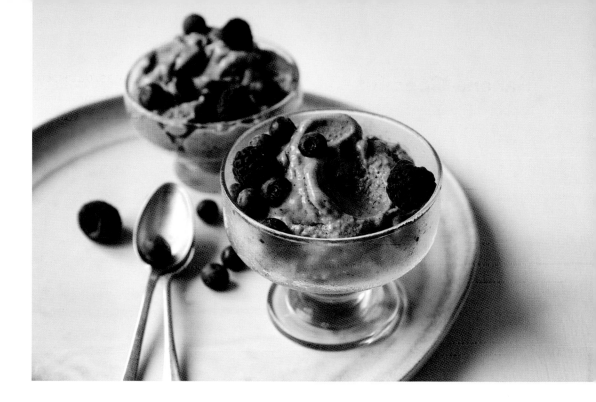

Very Berry Nice Cream

SERVES 2

PREP TIME: 10 minutes

PER SERVING: 270 calories, 7 g protein,
13 g fat, 31 g carbohydrates

---

2 frozen (very ripe) bananas, peeled
   before freezing

½ cup (60 g) frozen raspberries

½ cup (60 g) frozen blueberries

Scant ½ cup (100 ml) Almond Milk (page
   145)

2 tablespoons Almond Butter (page 150)

1 teaspoon Bourbon vanilla extract

½ teaspoon almond extract

Fresh berries

---

1. Blend the frozen bananas, raspberries,
and blueberries with the almond milk,
almond butter, vanilla, and almond extract
in a blender until creamy.

2. Divide between bowls. Top with fresh
berries and serve immediately.

Energy Balls

MAKES 12 BALLS
PREP TIME: 30 minutes
PER BALL: 150 calories, 4 g protein, 9 g fat,
13 g carbohydrates

---

7 ounces (200 g) Medjool dates, pitted
  (about 8)
1 cup (150 g) raw almonds
3 tablespoons Almond Butter (page 150)
2 teaspoons ground cinnamon
Cacao nibs

---

1. Soak the dates in warm water for 20
minutes, then drain.

2. Blend the almonds, almond butter, and
cinnamon in a blender until creamy. Add
the dates and blend into a smooth, sticky
dough.

3. Scoop out 1 tablespoon of the dough,
form into a ball, and roll in cacao nibs
until evenly coated. Repeat with the rest of
the dough.

4. Serve, or store the balls in the
refrigerator, where they will keep for up to
7 days.

Cashew-Coconut Balls

PER BALL: 125 calories, 2 g protein, 7 g fat,
14 g carbohydrates

Soak the same amount of dates as for the
Energy Balls, but blend them with ¾ cup
(100 g) cashews, ¼ cup (20 g) shredded
coconut, 2 tablespoons lime juice, and
1 tablespoon coconut oil. Roll the balls in
1 cup (80 g) shredded coconut.

Chocolate-Cardamom Balls

PER BALL: 140 calories, 4 g protein, 8 g fat,
12 g carbohydrates

Soak the same amount of dates as for
the Energy Balls, and blend them with
the same amount of almonds, but
add 2 tablespoons raw cacao powder,
1 teaspoon ground cardamom, and a
pinch of sea salt. Roll the balls in ground
hemp seeds.

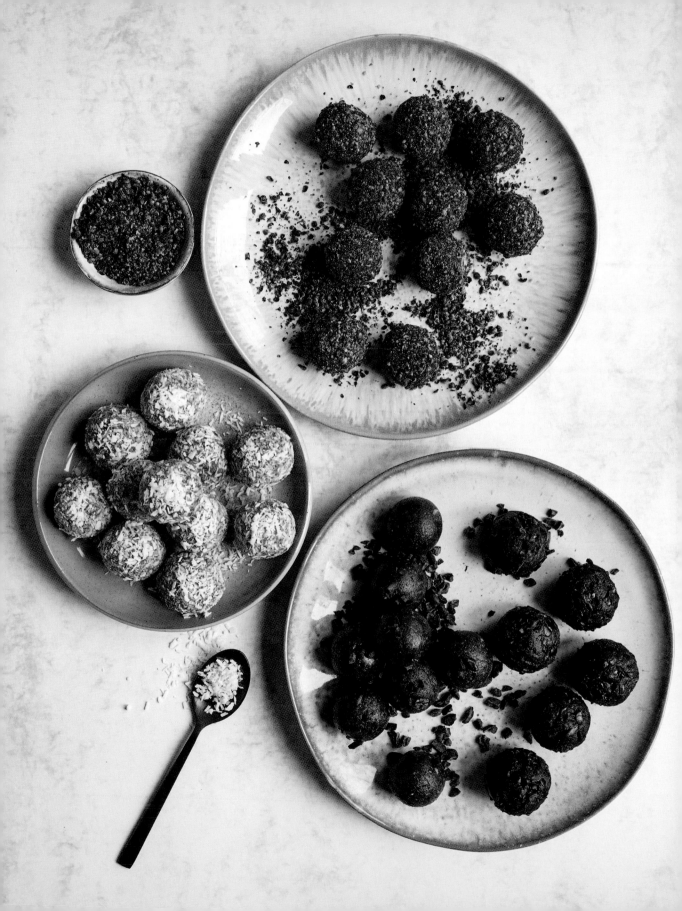

NOTES

1 Steven H. Woolf and Hedi Schoomaker, "Life Expectancy and Mortality Rates in the United States, 1959–2017," *JAMA* 322, no. 20 (2019): 1996–2016.

2 Jessica Y. Ho and Arun S. Hendi, "Recent Trends in Life Expectancy Across High Income Countries: Retrospective Observational Study," *BMJ* 362 (2018):k2562.

3 Michelle G. Kulovitz et al., "Potential Role of Meal Frequency as a Strategy for Weight Loss and Health in Overweight or Obese Adults," *Nutrition* 30, no. 4 (April 2014): 386–92.

4 J. A. Mattison et al., "Caloric Restriction Improves Health and Survival of Rhesus Monkeys," *Nature Communications* 8 (2017):14063.

5 Jaime Guevara-Aguirre et al., "Growth Hormone Receptor Deficiency Is Associated with a Major Reduction in Pro-Aging Signaling, Cancer, and Diabetes in Humans," *Science Translational Medicine* 3, no. 70 (February 2011): 70ra13.

6 Andrzej Bartke and John J. Kopchick, "The Forgotten Lactogenic Activity of Growth Hormone: Important Implications for Rodent Studies," *Endocrinology* 156, no. 5 (May 2015): 1620–22.

7 Tanya Zilberter, *Calorie Theories, Longevity, and Natural Health: The System of Dr. Shatalova and Current Discoveries* (2010).

8 Yifan Zhang et al., "The Effects of Calorie Restriction in Depression and Potential Mechanisms," *Current Neuropharmacology* 13, no. 4 (July 2015): 536–42.

9 Zhi-Lan Zhou et al., "Neuroprotection of Fasting Mimicking Diet on MPTP-Induced Parkinson's Disease Mice via Gut Microbiota and Metabolites," *Neurotherapeutics* 16, no. 3 (July 2019): 741–60.

10 Bae Kun Shin et al., "Intermittent Fasting Protects Against the Deterioration of Cognitive Function, Energy Metabolism and Dyslipidemia in Alzheimer's Disease-Induced Estrogen Deficient Rats," *Experimental Biology and Medicine* 243, no. 4 (February 2018): 334–43.

11 Tanya B. Dorff et al., "Safety and Feasibility of Fasting in Combination with Platinum-Based Chemotherapy," *BMC Cancer* 16, no. 360 (June 2016).

12 Stephan P. Bauersfeld et al., "The Effects of Short-Term Fasting on Quality of Life and Tolerance to Chemotherapy in Patients with Breast and Ovarian Cancer: A Randomized Cross-Over Pilot Study," *BMC Cancer* 18, no. 1 (December 2018): 476.

13 David A. Sinclair and Leonard Guarente, "Small-Molecule Allosteric Activators of Sirtuins," *Annual Review of Pharmacology and Toxicology* 54 (January 2014): 363–80.

14 Chia-Wei Cheng et al., "Prolonged Fasting Reduces IGF-1/PKA to Promote Hematopoietic-Stem-Cell-Based Regeneration and Reverse Immunosuppression," *Cell Stem Cell* 14, no. 6 (June 2014): 810–23.

15 Cheng et al., "Prolonged Fasting Reduces IGF-1/PKA."

16 Bodo C. Melnik, Swen Malte John, and Gerd Schmitz, "Over-Stimulation of Insulin/IGF-1 Signaling by Western Diet May Promote Diseases of Civilization: Lessons Learnt from Laron Syndrome," *Nutrition and Metabolism* 8 (June 2011): 41.

17 "Asthma," World Health Organization, who.int/news-room/q-a-detail/asthma.

18 James B. Johnson et al., "Alternate Day Calorie Restriction Improves Clinical Findings and Reduces Markers of Oxidative Stress and Inflammation in Overweight Adults with Moderate Asthma," *Free Radical Biology and Medicine* 42, no. 5 (March 2007): 665–74.

19 Matthew R. Alexander, "What Is the Global Prevalence of Hypertension (High Blood Pressure)?," medscape.com, updated February 22, 2019.

20 "More than 100 Million Americans Have High Blood Pressure, AHA Says," American Heart Association, accessed May 31, 2020, heart.org.

21 "Changes You Can Make to Manage High Blood Pressure," American Heart Association, updated November 30, 2017, heart.org.

22 "Diagnosed Diabetes, Total, Adults Aged 18+ Years, Age-Adjusted Percentage, National," United States Diabetes Surveillance System, Centers for Disease Control and Prevention, accessed June 5, 2020, gis.cdc.gov/grasp/diabetes/diabetesatlas.html.

23 "Migraine Facts," Migraine Research Foundation, accessed December 10, 2019, migraineresearchfoundation.org.

24 Allan Cott, "Controlled Fasting Treatment of Schizophrenia in the U.S.S.R." *Journal of Orthomolecular Medicine* 3, no. 1 (1971): 2–10.

25 Wenzhen Duan et al., "Brain–Derived Neurotrophic Factor Mediates an Excitoprotective Effect of Dietary Restriction in Mice," *Journal of Neurochemistry* 76, no. 2 (August 2008): 619–26.

26 Matthew C. L. Phillips, "Fasting as a Therapy in Neurological Disease," *Nutrients* 11, no. 10 (October 2019): 2501.

27 "Obesity and Overweight," World Health Organization, April 1, 2020, who.int.

28 Stephen C. Benoit et al., "Insulin and Leptin as Adiposity Signals," *Recent Progress in Hormone Research* 59 (2004): 267–85.

29 Aliki I. Venetsanopoulou et al., "Fasting Mimicking Diets: A Literature Review of Their Impact on Inflammatory Arthritis," *Mediterranean Journal of Rheumatology* 30, no. 4 (2019): 201–6.

30 J. Kjeldsen-Kragh et al., "Controlled Trial of Fasting and One-Year Vegetarian Diet in Rheumatoid Arthritis," *Lancet* 338, no. 8772 (October 1991): 899–902.

31 Marta Guasch-Ferré et al. "Meta-Analysis of Randomized Controlled Trials of Red Meat Consumption in Comparison with Various Comparison Diets on Cardiovascular Risk Factors," *Circulation* 139, no. 15 (April 2019): 1828–45.

32 Daniel Boffey, "Millions of Eggs Removed from European Shelves Over Toxicity Fears," *The Guardian,* August 3, 2017.

33 Erin L. Richman et al., "Egg, Red Meat, and Poultry Intake and Risk of Lethal Prostate Cancer in the Prostate-Specific Antigen-Era: Incidence and Survival," *Cancer Prevention Research* 4, no. 12 (December 2011): 2110–21.

34 Marcin Barański et al., "Effects of Organic Food Consumption on Human Health; the Jury Is Still Out!," *Food and Nutrition Research* 61, no. 1 (March 2017): 1287333.

35 Institute of Medicine, *Dietary Reference Intakes for Energy, Carbohydrate, Fiber, Fat, Fatty Acids, Cholesterol, Protein, and Amino Acids* (Washington, DC: National Academies Press, 2005).

36 Michael J. Shipton and Jecko Thachil, "Vitamin B_{12} Deficiency—A 21st Century Perspective," *Clinical Medicine* 15, no. 2 (April 2015): 145–50.

37 Shipton and Thachil, "Vitamin B_{12} Deficiency."

38 Ghanim Salih Mahdi, "The Atkin's Diet Controversy," *Annals of Saudi Medicine* 26, no. 3 (May–June 2006): 244–45.

39 "World Health Organization Says Processed Meat Causes Cancer," American Cancer Society, October 26, 2015, cancer.org.

40 "Processed Meats Increase Colorectal Cancer Risk, New Report," American Institute for Cancer Research, September 20, 2017, aicr.org.

41 Rashmi Sinha et al., "Meat Intake and Mortality: A Prospective Study of Over Half a Million People," *Archives of Internal Medicine* 169, no. 6 (March 2009): 562–71.

42 Bodo C. Melnik, Swen Malte John, and Gerd Schmitz, "Milk Is Not Just Food but Most Likely a Genetic Transfection System Activating mTORC1 Signaling for Postnatal Growth," *Nutrition Journal* 12, no. 1 (July 2013): 103.

43 Martijn J. C. van Herwijnen et al., "Abundantly Present MiRNAs in Milk-Derived Extracellular Vesicles Are Conserved Between Mammals," *Frontiers in Nutrition* 5 (September 2018): 81.

44 Van Herwijnen et al., "Abundantly Present MiRNAs in Milk-Derived Extracellular Vesicles."

45 Victor Gabriel Clatici et al., "Diseases of Civilization—Cancer, Diabetes, Obesity and Acne—the Implication of Milk, IGF-1 and mTORC1," *Maedica* 13, no. 4 (December 2018): 273–81.

46 K. Dahl-Jørgensen et al., "Relationship Between Cows' Milk Consumption and Incidence of IDDM in Childhood," *Diabetes Care* 14, no. 11 (November 1991): 1081–83.

47 Davaasambuu Ganmaa et al., "The Possible Role of Female Sex Hormones in Milk from Pregnant Cows in the Development of Breast, Ovarian and Corpus Uteri Cancers," *Medical Hypotheses* 65, no. 6 (2005): 1028–37.

Li-Qiang Qin et al., "Estrogen: One of the Risk Factors in Milk for Prostate Cancer," *Medical Hypotheses* 62, no. 1 (2004): 133–42.

Harald zur Hausen et al., "Dairy Cattle Serum and Milk Factors Contributing to the Risk of Colon and Breast Cancers," *International Journal of Cancer* 137, no. 4 (August 2015): 959–67.

48 Honglei Chen et al., "Consumption of Dairy Products and Risk of Parkinson's Disease," *American Journal of Epidemiology* 65, no. 9 (May 2007): 998–1006.

49 Bodo Melnik, "Milk Consumption: Aggravating Factor of Acne and Promoter of Chronic Diseases of Western Societies," *Journal of the German Society of Dermatology* 7, no. 4 (April 2009): 364–70.

50 Karl Michaëlsson, "Milk Intake and Risk of Mortality and Fractures in Women and Men: Cohort Studies," *BMJ* 349 (October 2014): g6015.

51 New Hampshire Department of Health and Human Services, *How Much Sugar Do You Eat? You May Be Surprised!*, dhhs.nh.gov /dphs/nhp/documents/sugar.pdf, August 2014.

52 L. Franzini et al., "Food Selection Based on High Total Antioxidant Capacity Improves Endothelial Function in a Low Cardiovascular Risk Population," *Nutrition, Metabolism & Cardiovascular Diseases* 22, no. 1 (January 2012): 50–57.

53 Vikas Kapil et al., "Dietary Nitrate Provides Sustained Blood Pressure Lowering in Hypertensive Patients: A Randomized, Phase 2, Double-Blind, Placebo-Controlled Study," *Hypertension* 65, no. 2 (February 2015): 320–27.

54 "Nonalcoholic Fatty Liver Disease," American Liver Foundation, accessed June 5, 2020, liverfoundation.org.

55 Lawrence K. Altman, "Three Americans Awarded Nobel for Discoveries of How a Gas Affects the Body," *The New York Times*, October 13, 1998.

56 Latika Sibal et al., "The Role of Asymmetric Dimethylarginine (ADMA) in Endothelial Dysfunction and Cardiovascular Disease," *Current Cardiology Reviews* 6, no. 2 (May 2010): 82–90.

57 H. Kahleova et al., "Vegetarian Diet Improves Insulin Resistance and Oxidative Stress Markers More Than Conventional Diet in Subjects with Type 2 Diabetes," *Diabetic Medicine* 28, no. 5 (May 2011): 549–59.

58 "Fat Consumption," Cancer Trends Progress Report, National Cancer Institute, updated March 2020, progressreport.cancer.gov /prevention/fat_consumption.

59 Kevin L. Fritsche, "The Science of Fatty Acids and Inflammation," *Advances in Nutrition* 6, no. 3 (May 2015): 293S–301S.

60 George A. Bray and Barry M. Popkin, "Dietary Fat Intake Does Affect Obesity!," *American Journal of Clinical Nutrition* 68, no. 6 (December 1998): 1157–73.

61 Julie A. Marshall and Daniel H. Bessesen, "Dietary Fat and the Development of Type 2 Diabetes," *Diabetes Care* 25, no. 3 (March 2002): 620–22.

62 Klaus G. Parhofer, "The Treatment of Disorders of Lipid Metabolism," *Deutsches Ärzteblatt International* 113, no. 15 (April 2016): 261–68.

63 "Can a Diet Give You Gout?" webmd.com, January 23, 2004.

64 Frank M. Sacks et al., "Dietary Fats and Cardiovascular Disease: A Presidential Advisory from the American Heart Association," *Circulation* 136, no. 3 (June 15, 2017): e1–e23.

65 Maryam Hussain et al., "High Dietary Fat Intake Induces a Microbiota Signature That Promotes Food Allergy," *Journal of Allergy and Clinical Immunology* 144, no. 1 (July 2019): 157–70.

66 Gabriel Fernandes, "Dietary Lipids and Risk of Autoimmune Disease," *Clinical Immunology and Immunopathology* 72, no. 2 (August 1994): 193–97.

67 R. L. Swank, "Multiple Sclerosis: Fat– Oil Relationship," *Nutrition* 7, no. 5 (September–October 1991): 368–76.

68 Martha Clare Morris and Christine C. Tangney, "Dietary Fat Composition and Dementia Risk," *Neurobiology of Aging* 35, no. S2 (September 2014): S59–S64.

69 Salk Institute, "Scientists Uncover How High-Fat Diet Drives Colorectal Cancer Growth," ScienceDaily, February 21, 2019, sciencedaily.com.

70 Sarah F. Brennan et al., "Dietary Fat and Breast Cancer Mortality: A Systematic Review and Meta-Analysis," *Critical Reviews in Food Science and Nutrition* 57, no. 10 (July 2017): 1999–2008.

71 NCI Staff, "Molecular Switch Links High- Fat Diet to Prostate Cancer Metastasis," National Cancer Institute, February 22, 2018, cancer.gov.

72 "Food Additive Status List," US Food and Drug Administration, updated October 24, 2019, fda.gov/food/food-additives-petitions /food-additive-status-list.

73 "Trans Fats," American Heart Association, reviewed March 23, 2017, heart.org.

74 "Trans Fats."

75 Jaime Uribarri et al., "Advanced Glycation End Products in Foods and a Practical Guide to Their Reduction in the Diet," *Journal of the American Dietetic Association* 110, no. 6 (June 2010): 911–16.

76 Claudia Luevano-Contreras and Karen Chapman-Novakofski, "Dietary Advanced Glycation End Products and Aging," *Nutrients* 2, no. 12 (December 2010): 1247–65.

77 Mary Jane Brown, "What Are Advanced Glycation End Products (AGEs)?," healthline.com, October 22, 2019.

78 Luevano-Contreras and Chapman-Novakofski, "Dietary Advanced Glycation End Products and Aging."

79 James A. King et al., "Incidence of Celiac Disease Is Increasing Over Time: A Systematic Review and Meta-Analysis," *American Journal of Gastroenterology* 115, no. 4 (April 2020): 507–25.

80 Ashley Marcin, "How Are Carbohydrates Digested?," healthline.com, updated June 27, 2019.

81 T. Momose, "Effect of Mastication on Regional Cerebral Blood Flow in Humans Examined by Positronic Tomography with ^{15}O-Labelled Water and Magnetic Resonance Imaging," *Archives of Oral Biology* 42, no. 1 (January 1997): 57–61.

82 Shawn Radcliffe and Stephanie Watson, "Overhydration: Types, Symptoms, and Treatments," healthline.com, updated March 7, 2019.

83 Wanda C. Reygaert, "Green Tea Catechins: Their Use in Treating and Preventing Infectious Diseases," *BioMed Research International* 2018 (July 2018): 9105261.

IMAGE CREDITS

SUBJECT INDEX

Page numbers in *italics* refer to photos.

Q

Quad Stretch + Knee Bend, 70, 70–71, 71
quinoa, 95

R

raw food, 93
recipes, daily, 101–2
See also separate recipe index
religious fasting, 13
rheumatism, 38–39
rice, 95
Rotation Stretches, 86, 86–87, 87

S

sea salt, 96
seeds, 95
self-healing, 10
serotonin, 21
sesame oil, 95
sesame seeds, 95
Shatalova, Galina, 16–17
Shoulder-Chest Stretch + Hip Dips, 84, 84–85, 85
Side Plank, 83, 83
simple sugars, 47
Sinclair, David A., 20
sirtuins, 20–21
Sit-Up, 69, 69
16:8 rule, 54–55
sleep, 22, 24
small intestine, 23
snacking, 56
spices, 96, 98
Spinal Stretch + Sit-Up, 68, 68–69, 69
stem cell production, 26
sugar, 47–50
sugar alternatives, 96
sugary foods, 92, 93
Superman, 75, 75

T

Tabletop, 81, 81
therapeutic fasting, 6–7
trans fats, 51
Tricep Stretch + Push-Up, 78, 78–79, 79
turmeric, 96

V

vegan diet, benefits of, 48–49
vegetables, 99, 100
vinegars, 95, 98
vitamin B$_{12}$, 44

W

walnuts, 95
water, 57–58
weekend, starting on, 90
Wendt, Lothar, 45
wheat, 52
white balsamic vinegar, 95
white wine vinegar, 95
wild rice, 95

RECIPE INDEX

Page numbers in *italics* refer to photos.

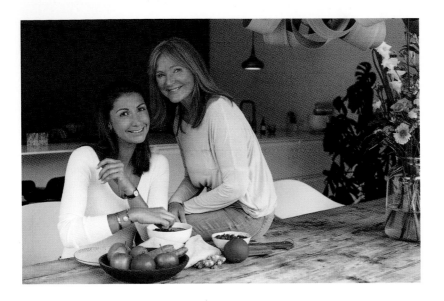

ABOUT THE AUTHORS

PETRA BRACHT is a general practitioner and specialist in natural healing—in particular, nutritional medicine—and the author of many bestselling books. She heads the first private vegan health center in Bad Homburg, Germany. Over the past thirty years, she has observed how even people with very severe diseases have been able to heal themselves through intermittent fasting and a plant-based diet. Her goal is that everyone become aware of how much they can do proactively to prevent disease and live a healthy life. She lives in Bad Homburg, Germany.

MIRA FLATT is a recipe developer who has worked intensively with Petra Bracht for the past eight years. She is a longtime vegan and has practiced intermittent fasting herself for the past six years. She lives in Bad Homburg, Germany.